Contents

Introduction v

1 Prenatal Concerns and Exercise Routine

Human Relations 2
Nutrition 2
Pregnancy Primer 4
Physiology 5
Before You Begin to Exercise 10
Guidelines for Running 11
Guidelines for Swimming 12
Guidelines for Strength Training 12
Using This Book at Home 13
Basic Exercise Positions 14
Breathing Exercises 17
Prenatal Exercise Routine 21

2 Focus on Delivery

Human Relations 71
Cesarean Delivery 71
Cesarean Preparation Exercises 72
Cesarean Delivery Hospital Exercises 78
Vaginal Delivery 83
Vaginal Delivery Hospital Exercises 84

3 Postpartum Concerns and Exercise Routine

Human Relations 91
Postpartum Exercise Routine 92

4 Postpartum Strength-training Routine

Introduction 135
Floor Exercises 136
Stationary Bicycle 136
Resistance Equipment 136

5 Focus on the Baby

Baby Massage 150
Patterning Your Baby's Reflexes 153
Exercises for Babies up to Four Months Old 154
Exercises for Babies Four to Twelve Months Old ... 167
Family Team Exercises 184
Make It Yourself 199

Appendix: Resources 201
Appendix: Pregnancy Primer 202
Index 205

Dedication

I dedicate this book to women everywhere who have the common goal of staying fit during pregnancy and who realize the necessity of getting back into shape after delivery and raising the healthiest babies possible.

To my family—husband Steve and sons Ryan and Reid—whose love and support I feel always. We share an interest in fitness throughout life and a family bond that brings special meaning to my life.

To Vivian Walrath, my grandmother, for sharing her knowledge, experience, and motivation.

Acknowledgments

This book is based on my original book, which included a foreword by Sandra Sackett, M.D.; an introduction by Rosalie Dauffenbach, R.N.; illustrations by John Boyer; and editing by Paul Kringle.

Special thanks to the members of the YMCA task force that helped me expand the "You & Me, Baby" program: Beth Dannhauser, Huntington, New York YMCA; Ellen Feeney-Pelliter, Eugene, Oregon YMCA; Colleen Kirby, Oklahoma City, Oklahoma YMCA; Terre Klipsch, Naperville, Illinois YMCA; Susan MacPhee, Portland, Maine YMCA; and Dr. Bill Zuti, YMCA of USA. Each of these capable people represents dozens of others who have been involved in classes on this subject.

Introduction

Exercises for Baby & Me is a book for any woman who is concerned about her own health and that of her baby. The exercise routines in the book were developed for use in YMCA fitness classes that are offered in hundreds of communities in the United States. These classes are for women who want to stay fit during pregnancy or get back into shape after delivery, and for parents of newborns who want to start their babies off on the road to fitness as a way of life.

Meadowbrook, Inc. is making this book available to thousands of pregnant women who may not know about the YMCA classes or who would prefer to do the exercise routines on their own. Whether you obtain this book from the YMCA, a bookstore, from a friend, or through a clinic or hospital program, please check with your medical caregiver to be sure he or she agrees with the information and suggestions presented here. There are many special circumstances that could influence what you should do before, during, or after your baby's birth.

Exercises for Baby & Me is based on the original work of Susan L. Regnier, which she self-published and, more importantly, shared, by training staff and volunteer leaders in local YMCAs across the country. Susan first developed the exercise routines for her own use during her first pregnancy and then taught others in the St. Paul Area YMCAs in Minnesota. In 1983, she brought together a task force of YMCA leaders, who had each developed programs for their communities, to expand the program and make it a national Y effort. This has resulted in a practical program that has been developed and tested for six years. The program has made a difference to literally thousands of women, whose participation and feedback to local YMCA staff have contributed to this book.

The contents of this book have been reviewed by Dr. Sandra Sackett, American Academy of Pediatrics and Twin City Obstetrics and Gynecology, LTD; and by Drs. John Brown, Jerome Scherek, John Farr, and Robert Braun. Still, there is no substitute for a thorough discussion between you and your doctor. Share this book with your doctor and ask specifically if she or he supports your engaging in the exercise routines suggested.

Exercises for Baby & Me is organized into five chapters. The first chapter discusses the changing human relationships in your life over the next nine months, principles of good nutrition during pregnancy, and basic physiological changes that occur during pregnancy. This discussion is followed by a summary of guidelines for running, swimming, and strength training. The chapter concludes with a detailed exercise routine that has been designed for and widely used by pregnant women across the country.

Chapter Two provides a set of exercises that can help you prepare for a cesarean delivery (many such deliveries are unexpected) and exercise routines for you to use in the hospital after delivery. Whether your delivery is vaginal or cesarean, the goal is still the same—a healthy baby.

Chapter Three takes up the issues of the postpartum period, including adjustments in family relationships and physical changes, and concludes with an effective exercise routine for getting back into shape.

Chapter Four presents a postpartum strength-training routine that includes a program of floor exercises, a stationary bicycle workout, and a resistance equipment (Nautilus and Universal) routine. The chapter concludes with a handy chart that outlines

INTRODUCTION

which muscle groups are exercised by which floor exercises and resistance machines.

Chapter Five focuses on your new baby. It introduces principles of massage and provides three different types of exercise routines: one for babies from birth to four months old, another for babies from four to twelve months old, and a third that will provide exercise for both you and your baby (including a few exercises that involve *both* parents as well as the baby). This chapter also includes practical sewing patterns to use in making your own exercise equipment.

In the appendix, you will find a list of resources—books, periodicals, and organizations—offering more information on specific topics. The appendix also includes a pregnancy primer that you may find helpful as various physiological problems and concerns arise. Again, this is not medical advice but basic information to help you understand possible causes and treatments. It is most important to see your doctor regularly throughout your pregnancy.

The "You & Me, Baby" program represents "wellness" in the most fundamental sense. The wellness concept suggests that:

- Each of us is responsible for our own health.
- Our health is a gift that we must work to maintain.
- To be well involves the whole person—body, mind, and spirit.
- We all need a support group—friends or relatives who care about how we feel and for whom we care in return.
- The quest for the full life is an ongoing, never-ending journey that brings both challenges and rewards every day!

The YMCA leadership and developers of the "You & Me, Baby" program wish you the greatest success in your journey.

Jerry Glashagel
National Consultant for Program Development
YMCA of the USA

Chapter One
Prenatal Concerns and Exercise Routine

The benefits of exercising during pregnancy are now widely accepted by medical and fitness specialists. Many prenatal caregivers prescribe exercise, in addition to the usual vitamins, in their prenatal care instructions. Firmer, better-toned muscles help you feel better, give you added strength in areas of your body stressed by pregnancy (particularly the back, abdomen, and pelvic area), and can make your delivery and postpartum recovery easier. Evidence in studies done by the Melpomene Institute of St. Paul, Minnesota, indicates that women who exercise when they are pregnant regain their shape sooner after pregnancy than women who do not.

The prenatal exercise routine on pages 21 to 70 is designed to keep you flexible and give you control over the degrees of strength and relaxation you need during delivery. As your baby grows, the difficulty of doing the exercises will increase. If the exercise routine doesn't seem strenuous at first, be patient and think of your priorities. This routine will maintain your strength, muscle tone, and flexibility while assuring your baby's overall well-being.

There are several ways to go about your regular exercise routine. Exercising by yourself at home offers the advantages of privacy and a flexible time schedule. On the other hand, you may prefer the opportunities for support and sharing of concerns that a group exercise class with other pregnant women can provide. An exercise class at the YMCA or another fitness center provides not only the advantage of mutual encouragement, but also the leadership of a trained person who will guide you through a routine of safe exercises and can help you find the answers to questions or concerns you may have.

Exercise can be done "on land"—indoors or outdoors—or in water, which is an ideal medium for exercise, especially for pregnant women. The buoyancy of your body in water promotes flexibility and allows you to move through a wide range of motions without danger of falling. Also, the resistance property of water demands a muscular effort, which serves as an effective toner for many parts of the body (e.g., arms and legs). The same property may also help prevent injuries since potentially harmful quick, jerky motions are less likely to occur in water.

The support of the water becomes increasingly helpful as you gain extra weight in the later months of your pregnancy. Exercise remains comfortable in the water when it might not on land, especially for exercises that involve the weight-bearing joints, such as the hips, knees, and ankles. Water exercise also helps control your body temperature and aids you in relaxing and cooling down. Many women find the YMCA swimming pools and water exercise programs ideal for their workouts during pregnancy. The Y is also a great place to join a prenatal exercise class "on land," in the gym or exercise area. Most Y prenatal exercise programs use the routine at the end of this chapter.

The rest of this introduction deals with human relations during pregnancy; nutritional needs of pregnant women; physiological changes (including changes in posture) that occur during pregnancy; and the cardiovascular system and its importance in preparing for

PRENATAL CONCERNS

labor and delivery. The chapter concludes with a description of basic exercise positions, breathing techniques, and the prenatal exercise routine.

Human Relations

Having a baby involves not just yourself, but a group of people—your partner, parents, grandparents, friends, perhaps other children, a doctor or midwife, and other members of the medical community. Each of these people affects how you feel. Your concerns about your own health and the health of your baby will be influenced by their reactions to your pregnancy and by the advice they offer you.

What you do about your health and fitness will, in turn, affect the lives of others. Exercise routines and eating habits, for example, are not strictly individual matters. Meals are generally important times for communicating as a family, and exercise and leisure activities often involve the whole family. How you get along with your partner, your friends, your relatives, and the new members of your private world from the medical community will make a difference in your social and mental health. During pregnancy, your attitude, which is highly influenced by your relationships with others, is a crucial component of your overall fitness.

The importance of developing and maintaining good relationships cannot be overemphasized. The three basic elements of good human relations are self-esteem, communication, and trust. During pregnancy, taking care of your mental health—by knowing what will make you feel good about yourself and by seeking those things out—is crucial to your self-esteem. In addition, your relationships with your medical caregivers, your husband, and others will benefit if you speak frankly about what you are thinking and feeling, and ask them to do the same. Finally, by respecting the rights of others to express themselves freely, you will help foster the mutual trust and respect that are vital to good communication and self-esteem.

Nutrition

Pregnancy is not the time to try the latest fad diets. Rather, it is a time to learn about and use principles of sound nutrition, since what you consume will affect both you and your baby. Learn as much about nutrition as you can so that you can plan what you eat. You needn't draw up menus to cover long periods of time—just keep in mind what you have on hand, how much time you have, and so on, to help you produce healthy, balanced meals. This may take some effort at first, but in time it will become second nature.

The major principle of good nutrition can be easily summed up: eat enough of what you need and not too much of what you don't need. But identifying what you do and don't need can be tricky, and applying that knowledge may be harder still. Fortunately, foods can be combined in an infinite number of ways to produce a healthful diet.

What does your body need? Food and water. More specifically, your body needs about fifty nutrients that it cannot manufacture for itself. Basically, these nutrients are proteins, vitamins, and minerals. Because no one food has all the nutrients you need, you should eat some of each of the four basic food types—protein suppliers, fruits and vegetables, grains, and milk and milk products—every day. Some foods fit into two categories—for example, milk and some legumes and grains are also good protein sources, and meat is a good source of iron, a mineral.

Protein Suppliers

Protein is made up of amino acids. Your body needs eight amino acids that it cannot produce itself.

PRENATAL CONCERNS

Complete protein is available from animal products—meat, fish, poultry, eggs, and milk. Grains, legumes (peas, beans, nuts), and seeds provide protein, but no grain, legume, or seed alone provides a complete protein. However, they can be mixed or combined with milk or cheese to provide protein as complete as that available in animal products. For example, peanut butter on whole wheat bread, beans and rice, and oatmeal and milk work complimentarily to produce complete protein.

Fruits and Vegetables

Fruits and vegetables provide minerals and vitamins, carbohydrates for your body to burn, and fiber for better digestion. Processing and preparation affect the nutritional value of these foods; for example, heat causes some vitamins, particularly vitamin C, to break down. Fresh, raw vegetables provide the most nutrition; other forms of preparation provide less. The blanching and heat sealing involved in the commercial canning of vegetables can significantly decrease their nutritional worth.

Cereals

Cereals include whole and enriched grains, rice, bread, noodles, and spaghetti. They supply protein, carbohydrates, fiber, vitamins, and minerals.

Milk and Milk Products

This food group includes milk, cheese, yogurt, and cottage cheese. Milk and milk products are good sources of calcium, vitamin D, and protein.

Special Issues

Within the context of the principles of sound nutrition are several special issues related to pregnancy. One of these issues has to do with how much you eat. A common problem in the first three months of pregnancy is lack of appetite, often accompanied by vomiting. This is the time to talk with your caregiver about food supplements or vitamins. He or she may suggest supplements to make up for nutrients not eaten or lost through vomiting. You may also need to compensate for an overall lack of calories.

Do not take food supplements or vitamins during your pregnancy without first checking with your doctor.

Basic Food Group Servings

The Proteins Group

Recommended minimum during pregnancy: Three to four servings per day.

What is a serving?

1 small chicken leg
1/2 small chicken breast
2 slices of chicken, turkey, veal, lamb, liver, beef, ham, or pork
1 hamburger patty
2 eggs
1/2 cup cottage cheese
2 slices of cheddar cheese
1 cup cooked beans or lentils, combined with rice, macaroni, or bread
4 T. peanut butter and one slice of bread

The Fruits and Vegetables Group

Recommended minimum during pregnancy: Four servings per day.

What is a serving?

1 cup raw salad (excluding dressing)
1/2 cup cooked fruit or vegetables
1 medium cantaloupe
1/2 cup berries
10-12 grapes or cherries
1/2 medium banana or grapefruit
2 medium plums, nectarines
1 medium pear, orange, apple
6 oz. unsweetened fruit juice

The Breads and Cereals Group

Recommended minimum during pregnancy: Four servings per day.

What is a serving?

1 slice of bread
1/2 - 3/4 cup cooked cereal
1 roll, biscuit or muffin
1 oz. (about 1 cup) ready-to-eat cereal
1/2 - 3/4 cup cooked macaroni, spaghetti, or noodles

The Milk Group

Recommended minimum during pregnancy: Four servings per day.

What is a serving?

1 cup milk
1 slice of Swiss cheese
1 cup yogurt
1 cup custard
1 cup cottage cheese

PRENATAL CONCERNS

Typical Weight Gain Distribution During Pregnancy	
Placenta	1.4 lbs.
Uterus	2.0 lbs.
Blood	4.0 lbs.
Baby	7.7 lbs.
Amniotic Fluid	1.8 lbs.
Breast Tissue	0.9 lbs.
Tissue Fluid	2.7 lbs.
Other	3.5 lbs.
TOTAL	24.0 lbs.

Excessive amounts of some vitamins, such as A and D, can harm your baby. On the other hand, all of your nutrient needs are greater during pregnancy, and the need for iron is nearly impossible to meet without a supplement. Your caregiver may recommend supplements to increase your intake of iron and other vitamins and minerals.

The issue of how much weight you can expect to gain safely with appropriate eating should be answered by your doctor. The chart at left lists some of the common weight-gain categories for a woman who gained twenty-four pounds on the way to delivering a seven-pound, seven-ounce baby.

Other Health Concerns

There are several other *don'ts* related to substances that can be particularly dangerous to good health during pregnancy:

- *Don't smoke.* Current research suggests that smoking during pregnancy is associated with low birth weight and with an increase of miscarriages and stillbirths. You should also avoid contact with smokers as much as possible, since there is increasing evidence that sidestream smoke is unhealthy for those who inhale it. In fact, the people who breathe in the smoke from another person's cigarette can ingest more of several harmful smoke by-products than the smoker does.

- *Don't drink alcoholic beverages.* In a number of ways, alcohol can pose a threat to the unborn baby. Alcohol can interfere with the normal growth process of fetal cells. The percentage of alcohol in the bloodstream of the developing baby is the same as the percentage of alcohol in the mother's bloodstream.

- *Cut down on or eliminate caffeine.* The caffeine in coffee, tea, cola drinks, chocolate, and many over-the-counter medications stimulates the central nervous system. The use of caffeine can be related to nervousness, restlessness, insomnia, and heartburn. Current research is also investigating the possible relationship between consumption of large amounts of caffeine and birth defects. The safe thing to do is to cut out caffeine altogether during pregnancy.

- *Don't take any medication or drug without first discussing it with your doctor.* Aspirin, antihistamines, sleeping aids, and, for some people, marijuana and other drugs have become part of everyday life. Because these substances can influence the early development of the baby, it is advisable to discontinue use of all medications and drugs, especially during the first three months of pregnancy. If you feel you need any medication, talk to your doctor to see what he or she recommends.

Conclusion

Pregnancy is a time to eat a balanced diet of healthy foods and to feel good as a result. A feeling of vitality comes from eating just enough of a variety of foods from the four basic groups. Feeling good never comes from overeating, or from consuming large quantities of fats and of high-calorie goodies. Your pregnancy is a perfect time to explore truly good eating habits and to discover the pleasures of feeling really good when you eat correctly!

Pregnancy Primer

The pregnancy primer on pages 202 to 204 lists fourteen problems commonly associated with pregnancy (e.g., nausea, varicose veins, stretch marks), together with possible causes and solutions. However, this information should by no means be considered a substitute for a discussion with your medical caregiver about any physiological or psychological concerns you have during your pregnancy.

PRENATAL CONCERNS

Physiology

A number of changes occur in your body during pregnancy; there are new feelings and, sometimes, discomforts to contend with. And the final act of labor is plain hard work. You will find each stage of pregnancy more manageable if you understand what is going on in your body and if you work to keep your muscles and your entire cardiovascular system in the best possible condition.

Several major changes in your physiology occur during pregnancy:

- Your uterus increases in size to accommodate the growing baby. As it stretches it may cause some discomfort in your internal ligament support structures.
- Your uterus, which is located in the pelvic cavity bordered in back by the spinal column, is pushed forward into the abdominal wall as it increases in size.
- Your vagina and birth canal are supported by the pelvic floor musculature. As your uterus enlarges, your vagina is subjected to pressure.
- Your gastrointestinal system can be upset as a result of pressure on and displacement of your stomach and intestines as your uterus enlarges.
- Your breasts usually increase in size and become tender.
- Your blood volume can increase by 30 to 50 percent, and your heart rate may increase an average of ten to fifteen beats per minute. Generally blood pressure does not increase despite the increase in blood volume and heart rate.
- Your respiratory system is affected in two ways. Your lung capacity may be reduced as your uterus enlarges and your diaphragm moves up. Also, hormones released during pregnancy can cause your body to be more sensitive to carbon dioxide, resulting in an increased likelihood of rapid fatigue from vigorous activity.

There is little, if anything, you can do to prevent breast tenderness or discomfort caused by the stretching of the ligaments of your uterus. However, you can reduce some of the other major physiological discomforts by doing specific exercises to strengthen your pelvic floor and abdominal muscles, and by performing regular exercise to keep your cardiovascular system in good shape. These exercises and cardiovascular concerns are discussed in the following pages.

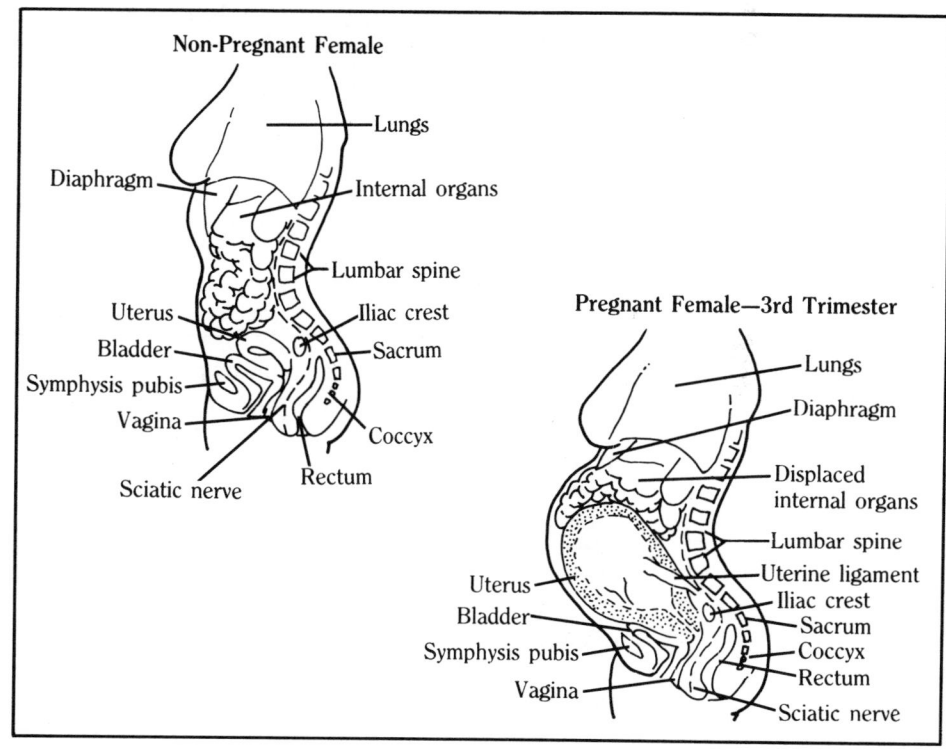

PRENATAL CONCERNS

Pelvic Floor Musculature and the Kegel Exercise

In preparing for delivery, it is important that you understand the pelvic floor musculature and practice the "kegel" exercise, which involves contracting your pelvic floor muscles. The exercise was named for Dr. Arnold Kegel, one of the first physicians to stress the importance of the pelvic floor musculature.

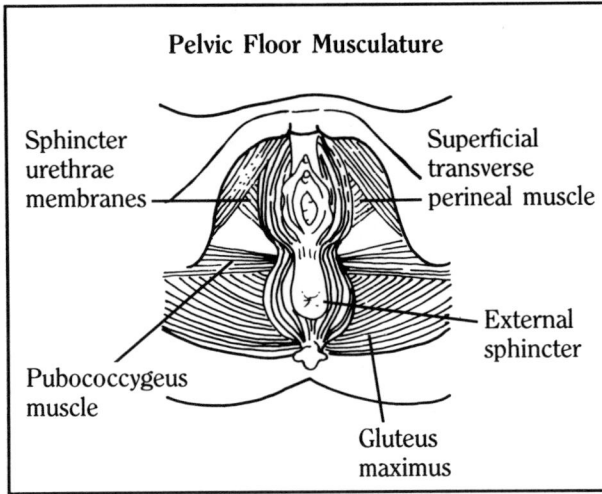

The hammocklike pelvic floor (or perineal) muscles, which stretch from your pubic bone to your tailbone (coccyx), support your pelvic organs such as the uterus, bladder, and bowel. Your pelvic floor also relaxes and contracts when you urinate. During pregnancy, your pelvic floor muscles may sag in response to hormonal changes and the increasing weight of your uterus.

Because the condition of the pelvic floor muscles is of lifelong importance, doing the kegel exercise regularly is essential both during pregnancy and throughout your lifetime. Among the many benefits of maintaining the muscle tone of your pelvic floor are increased support of your pelvic organs and better bladder control. Long-term benefits include proper positioning of your internal organs within your pelvic area.

To become aware of the muscles you are exercising when you "kegel," try to stop the flow of urine as you urinate. (You may practice in this fashion while you are learning to kegel, but you should not use this method continuously.)

The kegel exercise can be done in any position. Think of the pelvic floor as an elevator. Contract your pelvic floor muscles a little at a time, as if you are going up the floors from ground to fifth floor. Hold the muscles tightly at the top, then slowly release them as you descend to the ground floor. When you arrive at the ground floor, think "release" to try to relax the muscles even further. This should be done smoothly and gradually. Do not hold your breath while you are doing the kegel exercise.

Kegels can be done during intercourse with your partner, who can give you feedback on how you are doing. As an added bonus, your kegels may enhance your partner's sexual response. You should start doing kegels now, do them throughout your pregnancy, do a kegel or relax your pelvic floor during labor and pushing, and continue to do kegels after delivery to promote healing of your perineum and to restore your pelvic floor to its original tone and keep it that way.

Recti Diastasis

During pregnancy, you may experience some degree of recti diastasis, or separation of the abdominal muscles. Especially in the second trimester of pregnancy, your abdominal (rectus) muscles are susceptible to the internal pressure exerted by your uterus as the baby pushes from within it. The structure of the female abdominal muscles make it possible for them to separate at the center seam (linea alba) that runs vertically down the middle of your abdomen.

PRENATAL CONCERNS

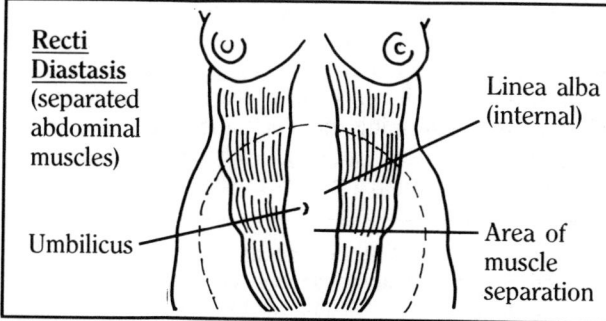

Recti Diastasis (separated abdominal muscles)
Umbilicus
Linea alba (internal)
Area of muscle separation

Posture

Another important physiologic concern during pregnancy is posture. Your posture will change dramatically and quickly as your uterus enlarges and your abdominal muscles are stretched to capacity. The strain is felt on your distended abdomen and in the increased lumbar (low back) spinal curve. Your spine, particularly in the lumbar region, becomes an anchor that compensates for the gradual shift in your center of gravity. As the abdominal distension and spinal curvature increase, you may begin to lean back on your heels, thereby further increasing the lumbar curve. This "swaybacked" posture will, in turn, tend to increase the likelihood and severity of lower back pain.

Poor posture is generally caused by a lack of integrity of the abdominal and gluteal (buttock) muscles. When your abdominal and gluteal muscles are working together to keep your pelvis positioned properly, your spine can keep your head and shoulders in proper alignment. If your gluteal muscles are tight, your quadriceps (thigh muscles) will relax, which in turn will keep your knees from hyperextending. Your feet will then be

Separation of the abdominal muscles is caused by a combination of hormonal changes, excessive strain, and sudden jerking movements. It is important that you regain the stability and integrity of separated abdominal muscles by performing specific abdominal exercises as soon as possible after delivery.

The exercises in this book are intended to help you maintain and regain the strength and tone of your abdominal muscles. However, before beginning any of the exercise routines, have your doctor check for abdominal muscle separation, or use the self-test below.

1. Lie on your back with your knees bent, your heels by your hips.
2. Place your fingertips on your abdomen, on the soft tissue area just above your navel. Use your navel as a "landmark" to keep your fingertips in place.
3. Pull your chin to your chest and curl your shoulders off the floor while pressing firmly on your abdomen with your fingers.
4. Feel for the tautness of the muscle bands and gauge the size of the soft region between these bands. Any width greater than approximately one inch should be treated with caution, and indicates that you should progress gradually in the degree of difficulty for the abdominal exercises in this book.

Self-Test for Separation of the Abdominal Muscles
(Recti Diastasis)

PRENATAL CONCERNS

better able to support your added body weight without being forced to point outward in the so-called "pregnant waddle."

Your pelvis, which supports your spinal column, takes on an important role in your posture during pregnancy. The increasing weight of your uterus and stretching of your uterine wall will cause your pelvis to tend to angle forward. Therefore, it is especially important during pregnancy that you keep your pelvis tilted back in order to maintain good posture and minimize lumbar curve. Performing the Tuck and Pull exercise (below), which involves "tucking" your pelvis in and pulling in your abdominal muscles, will help you do so.

Tuck and Pull Exercise

Practicing this exercise whenever possible will help promote good posture during pregnancy. The movements you perform in doing the exercise precede many specific prenatal and postnatal exercises. Learn to move smoothly through the exercise so that the individual actions "flow" as a natural movement.

In this exercise, the muscles of your trunk work together to perform the pelvic tilt (tuck):

1. Stand with your knees unlocked and slightly bent. "Tuck" your pelvis in and pull in your abdominal muscles (this allows for a pelvic rocking action).
2. Contract your secondary abdominal muscles and buttocks (this allows your diaphragm to expand and flattens your lower back).

The Cardiovascular System

Because the maternal circulatory system is the source of fetal oxygen and nutrition, the condition of your heart and lung (cardiovascular) system during pregnancy makes a difference in the amount of oxygen-rich blood your baby will receive. The condition of this system will improve with regular exercise. If you have been exercising regularly, being pregnant is no reason to quit. On the contrary, it is a good reason to continue. If you have not been working out, now is the time to start!

An important component of the cardiovascular portion of the workout is monitoring your target heart rate. Your target heart rate is the rate at which your heart ideally should be beating during the part of the workout—walking or jogging, for example—when your body demands, produces, and distributes more oxygen than usual over a sustained period of time (generally, twenty to thirty minutes).

The target heart rate training zone chart on page 9 shows the normal target-heart-rate range by age, and a special pregnancy target-heart-rate range (also by age), which is slightly below the normal target range. It is important to work up to the level of the lower number, but not higher than the higher number, and to sustain that workload for twenty to thirty minutes.

PRENATAL CONCERNS

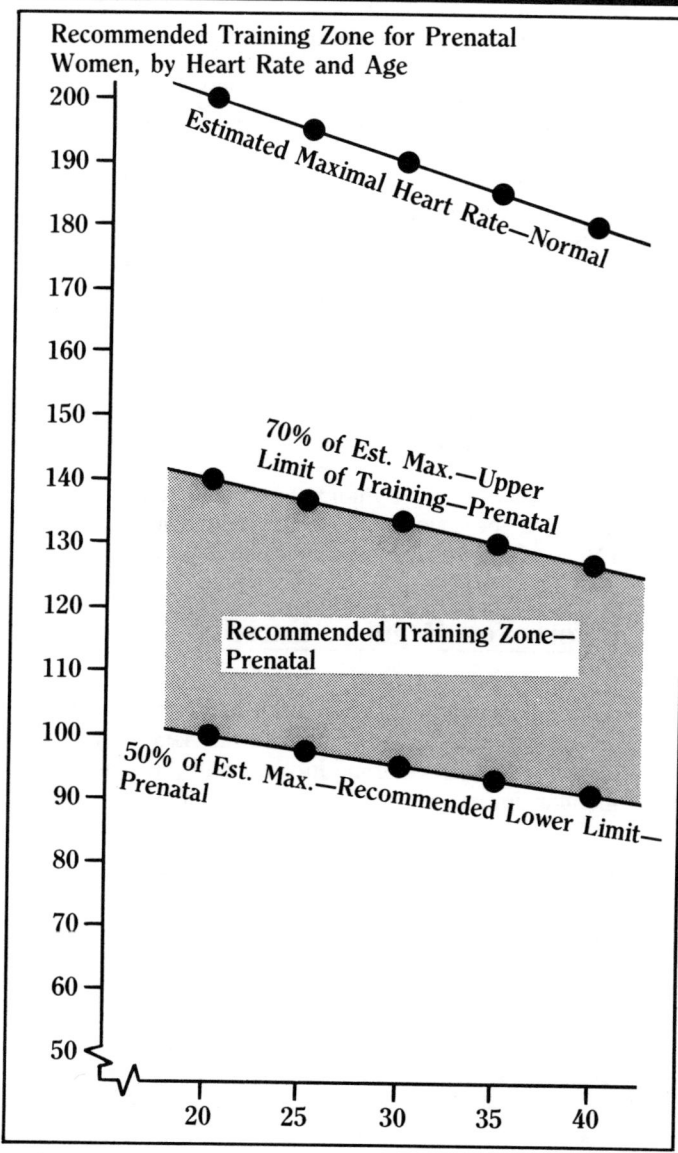

Recommended Training Zone for Prenatal Women, by Heart Rate and Age

Predicted Maximal 70% and 50% Heart Rate by Age

Age	Predicted Max	70% (60 sec.)	50% (60 sec.)
20	200	140	100
21	199	139	
22	198	139	99
23	197	138	
24	196	138	98
25	195	137	
26	194	136	97
27	193	135	
28	192	134	96
29	191	134	
30	190	133	95
31	189	132	
32	188	131	94
33	187	131	
34	186	130	93
35	185	129	
36	184	128	92
37	183	128	
38	182	127	91
39	181	126	
40	180	126	90
41	179	125	
42	178	125	89
43	177	124	
44	176	123	88
45	175	123	

Conversion of Heart Rate (bpm) to 10 Second Count

Maximal Heart Rate	70% (10 sec.)	50% (10 sec.)	Age
200	23		20
199	"		21
198	"		22
197	"		23
196	"		24
195	"		25
194	"		26
193	"		27
192	22	16	28
191	"		29
190	"		30
189	"		31
188	"		32
187	"		33
186	"		34
185	"		35
184	21		36
183	"		37
182	"		38
181	"		39
180	"	15	40
179	"		41
178	"		42
177	"		43
176	"		44
175	20		45

Source: Astrand, modification based on 220 − Age = Max HR

PRENATAL CONCERNS

To determine your target heart rate:

1. Press the fingertips of your right hand firmly into your left wrist, just below your left thumb. Do *not* use your thumb to take your pulse; it has a pulse of its own.

2. Take your pulse, using a watch or clock with a second hand as you count the beats.

3. Count the pulse beats for ten seconds and multiply by six for a minute count; or take a six-second count and multiply by ten.

4. Use the target-heart-rate chart to find your ideal target-heart-rate range.

5. If you choose not to use the chart, you can use the following formula: Take your age and subtract it from 220 to find your maximum heart rate. Your target-heart-rate range is fifty to seventy percent of your maximum heart rate. *Example:* If you are 30 years old, calculate your target-heart-rate range as follows:

220 − 30 (age) = 190 (Maximum Heart Rate)
.50 × 190 = 95
.70 × 190 = 133
Target-heart-rate range = 95 (lower level) to 133 (upper level)

Take your pulse at the beginning, middle, and end of the cardiovascular portion of your exercise workout—e.g., before and after walking or jogging—and check your heart rate at the very end of your workout. Your pulse should be between sixteen and eighteen beats, or lower, in a ten-second count. If it is higher than eighteen beats, be sure to continue to cool down until you are within this range. Never work up to your maximum heart rate.

If you want more information about target heart rates, ask the trained fitness leaders at your local YMCA or another physical fitness organization.

Before You Begin to Exercise

Remember that many prenatal exercises can be done in water as well as on land. In the prenatal exercise routine (pages 21 to 70), the name of any exercise that can be done in water with little or no modification is followed by a water symbol:

Before you begin the prenatal exercise routine, you'll want to review these general principles of sound exercise programs:

• Check with your doctor before starting an exercise program. You should be healthy and have no complicating medical problems before starting such a program. Look over the exercises in this book, and then consult your doctor to make sure there are no reasons why you should not do any of them.

PRENATAL CONCERNS

- Check for separation of your abdominal muscles, using the self-test on page 7, or have your doctor check to see whether you should take care in doing (or avoid doing) any of the exercises designed to strengthen and maintain the tone of your abdominal muscles.

- During the first three months of pregnancy, monitor your body temperature when exercising. It is important that you not raise the core body temperature above 100 degrees F. during this period, since the developing baby does not yet have the ability to dissipate body heat. Thus, avoid overexercising in a hot environment or otherwise raising your body temperature.

- Begin your exercise routine slowly, taking care to do the warm-up exercises first. Do easy stretching and loosening-up exercises before engaging in cardiovascular exercise.

- If a position in any exercise is uncomfortable, adjust to a similar position that feels more comfortable.

- The suggested number of repetitions for each exercise is only a recommendation; you may want to do fewer or more than the number specified, depending on your fitness level.

- If you feel a strain or pain of any kind, stop exercising and rest for a few moments. The next time you try that exercise, remember to take it easy.

- To get the maximum benefit from the exercise routine, do as much of each exercise as possible, do as many exercises in the routine as you can, and follow the order in which the exercises are given.

- Follow exercising with a cool-down period. A simple cool-down routine will help you begin to relax, get your heart rate back to normal, and allow your muscles to comfortably return to their unstretched state.

- Take your pulse at the beginning, middle, and end of the cardiovascular portion of the routine. Then check your recovery heart rate at the very end of your workout. (For information on target heart rate, see pages 8 to 10.)

Guidelines for Running

- Heat and dehydration can be serious problems. Run during the coolest part of the day, and wear appropriate clothing. Be sure to drink plenty of fluids before a run, even if you may have problems with urinary frequency.

- Wear comfortable clothing. Well-cushioned, stable running shoes and a good bra are especially important.

- Be kind to your back. Pay attention to your posture and balance. Experiment with posture changes that make you more stable while running. Some women find that a lightweight maternity girdle offers support for their back and ligaments. And maternity support stockings also help some women feel more comfortable.

- Take the time for adequate warm-up and cool-down, before and after running.

- Be willing to modify your runs in terms of intensity, frequency, and speed. As you advance through your pregnancy, increasing weight and fatigue may dictate shorter, slower runs, eliminating hills and speed work.

- Don't be afraid to stop and walk. This may be necessary due to heat, ligament or joint pains, or Braxton-Hicks contractions.

- Run with others, if possible. And always let people know when and where you are running. Bring money in case you need to call for a ride home.

PRENATAL CONCERNS

Guidelines for Swimming

- Be sure the water and air temperatures are comfortable. Leave the water if you feel too chilled or overheated.

- Wear a comfortable suit. Some maternity suits may become too heavy when wet and make swimming difficult. Experiment with different styles and sizes until you find something that gives you the necessary support and comfort.

- Take time to warm up. Try doing some stretching on land or in the water. Start off swimming slowly until you loosen up.

- Swim according to your abilities. And use moderation in setting the frequency, length, and pace of your workouts.

- If you experience contractions, leg cramps, or joint pains, be ready to stop swimming or change your swimming style. For instance, try different strokes, kicks, or turns.

- Modify or stop your exercise program if medical conditions make it necessary (for instance, due to early dilation or bag of water leaking).

- Do not swim alone, in case you get cramps. But try to avoid crowds; if you swim more than two in a lane, you might get kicked or hit accidentally.

- Diving or jumping into the water feet first, as well as water skiing, are not recommended.

Guidelines for Strength Training

- Strength training is recommended only for those women who are free of any medical complications with their pregnancy and who have no current problems with muscle, bone, or joint injury.

- Work up to a comfortable pressure or weight, and maintain a regular strength-training routine.

- Do up to twelve repetitions slowly; stop when you feel "muscle burn" or any pain or discomfort. If you can do twelve repetitions easily, increase the pressure/weight slightly, following the principles of stress adaptation.

- Do abductor/adductor exercises only if they feel comfortable.

- Omit hip and back exercises after your fourth month of pregnancy. Also omit these exercises if you have a bad back.

- When using the overhead press machine, use only light pressure or weight.

- Emphasize the development of your laterals and shoulders. This is especially important during later pregnancy, when the shoulders start to drop to compensate for the added weight of the baby.

- Avoid holding your breath, which causes unnecessary blood pressure elevation. Exhale during the lifting or exerting phase, and inhale during the lowering or negative resistance phase.

- To supplement your workout, try a twenty- to thirty-minute walk. Or add a ten- to fifteen-minute cardiovascular stationary bicycle ride or lifecycle workout before using the resistance equipment.

Machines to Use

- Leg extension
- Hip abductor/adductor
- Pullover torso*
- Rowing torso
- Double-chest*
- Lateral raise
- Biceps
- Triceps

*Receive instruction before trying this machine on your own.

PRENATAL CONCERNS

Machines to Use with Caution

- Hip/back (stop at fourth month)
- Overhead press (with light weight only)
- Hip flexor
- Neck and shoulder
- Four-way neck
- Torso arm pulldown
- Rotary neck (prefer four-way neck machine)

Machines to Avoid

- Hip/back (after fourth month and altogether if you have a lower-back or sciatica problem)
- Squat
- Leg curl
- Compound leg
- Lower-back
- Abdominal
- Multiexercise

Note: If you have back problems, also avoid the rotary torso, overhead press, and hip/back machines.

Postpartum Women

After receiving your doctor's approval, follow a beginner's general workout. Use the abductor/adductor machines with caution. Also, start out very slowly, using low pressure and weight, especially with the lower-back and abdominal machines.

See Chapter 4 on strength training for postpartum women.

Using This Book at Home

If you are using this book on your own, rather than in conjunction with a You & Me, Baby exercise class, you'll benefit most from the prenatal exercise routine if you perform it at least three times a week.

The exercises are intended to be performed in the order in which they are presented here. Be sure to read the instructions above in "Before you Begin to Exercise" before beginning the exercise routine.

BASIC POSITIONS

Sitting Positions

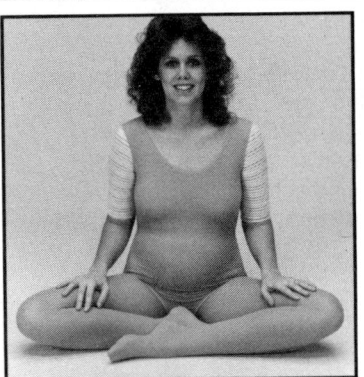

Tailor Sit
Sit tall and fold your legs comfortably in front of your body.

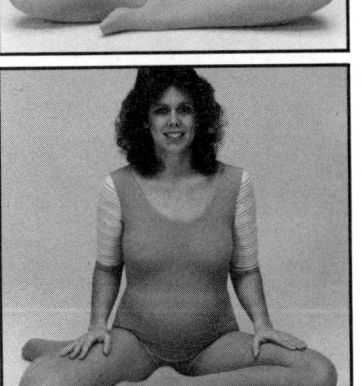

Side Sit
Sit tall, with both your knees bent, so that the bottom of your left foot touches the inside of your right thigh, and your right heel touches your right buttock (or reverse the leg positions).

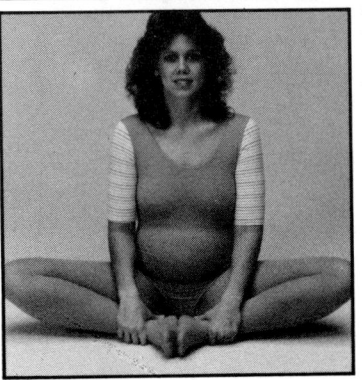

Butterfly Sit
Sit tall with the soles of your feet touching.

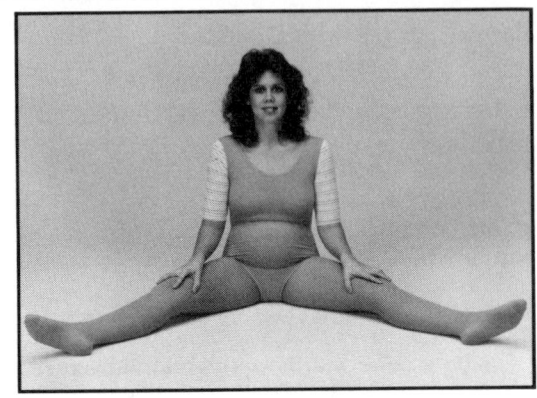

Straddle Sit
Sit tall and extend your legs in front of your body in a V position.

Pike Sit
Sit tall and extend your legs directly in front of your body so that your body forms an L.

BASIC POSITIONS

Arm Positions

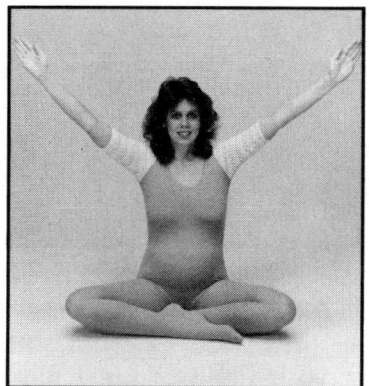

V Position
Extend your arms overhead in a V.

Cross Position
Extend your arms out to your sides at shoulder level.

Feet Positions

Feet Flexed
Sit tall and extend your legs in front of you with your feet perpendicular to the floor. Sitting as tall as possible, flex feet (toes pointing upward).

Toes Pointed
Sit tall and extend your legs in front of you, pointing your toes straight out from your body.

BASIC POSITIONS

Body Positions

All Fours
Roll over to your hands and knees. Strive to keep your body balanced so that your shoulders are aligned with your flat palms and your hips are aligned with your knees.

Back Tuck
Lie flat on your back and draw both knees into your chest or around your belly. Keep your back flat on the floor.

Hook-Lying
Lie flat on your back with your knees bent and your feet flat on the floor.

Rolling to a Standing Position

1 Whenever you move from a lying position to a standing position when you are pregnant, begin by rolling onto your side. Place the palm of your hand flat on the floor to gently raise your upper body, then gradually roll to your knees.

2 Once you are on all fours, place your feet flat on the floor, one at a time.

3 To straighten up from a forward-leaning position (i.e., upper body hanging loosely), bend your knees so that your thigh muscles can assist in lifting your upper body weight. When your upper body is straight, straighten your knees to stand.

BREATHING EXERCISES

Because proper breathing helps you to relax and relieves tension, it can help during labor as well as when you exercise. When you do the exercises in the prenatal and post-partum routines, inhale as you relax and exhale as you hold a stretch or isometric contraction.

The following breathing exercises are most beneficial when done during a warm-up or cool-down routine, or whenever you need to relax. To do the exercises properly, keep your spine straight and your eyes open, and clear your mind of everything but your breathing. Breathe slowly, quietly, and continuously, taking air in through your nose to purify it. Work up gradually to a comfortable limit of air; taking in too much air can cause over-oxidation and hyperventilation or dizziness.

Simple Breath

Aim: To teach you to breathe down into your diaphragm.

Starting Position: Tailor sit, with your hands on your stomach and the fingertips of your middle fingers touching lightly.

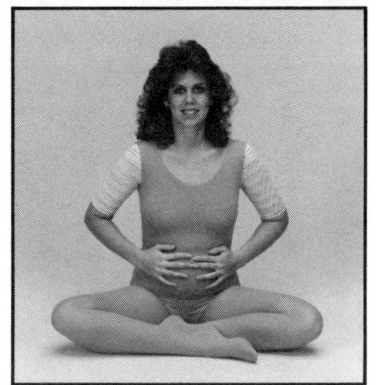

1. Breathing in through your nose, bring air into your lungs and allow it to push your stomach outward. Your fingertips should move apart slightly as your stomach expands. Hold your breath for a count of five, then slowly exhale (this will bring your fingertips back together). *Repetitions:* Repeat slowly three to four times.

Swan Breath

Aim: To teach you to breathe with your body movements and to expand your rib cage, giving your heart more room to work in.

Starting Position: Straddle sit, with your arms at your sides.

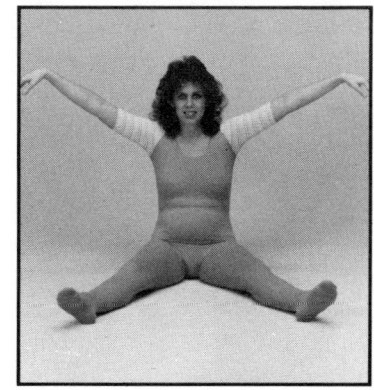

1. Bring your arms into cross position, inhaling through your nose as you move your arms upward. Exhale through your mouth while bringing your arms down. *Repetitions:* Repeat three to four times.

17

BREATHING EXERCISES

Sniffing and Vitalic Breath

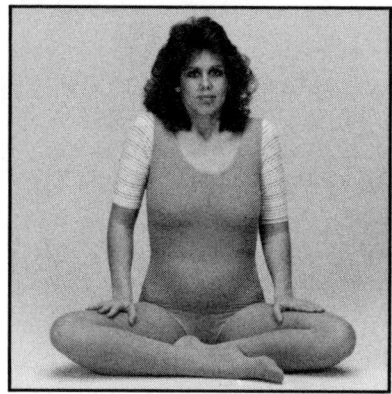

Aim: To cleanse and strengthen your lungs (many pregnant women have trouble breathing from cold and allergy symptoms).

Starting Position: Tailor sit.

1 Breathe a series of sharp sniffs through your nose until your lungs are completely full, then blow the air out sharply through your mouth, with a loud "HAAA." *Repetitions:* Repeat three to four times.

Alternate Nostril Breathing

Aim: To create a natural tranquilizing effect, calm your nervous system, and clear your sinuses.

Starting Position: Tailor sit.

Note: No one with high blood pressure or heart problems should hold her breath. You can, however, still benefit from this exercise by inhaling in one nostril and exhaling immediately out the other. Do not hold both nostrils closed.

1 With the middle fingers of your right hand between your eyebrows, place your right thumb on your right nostril and your little finger on your left nostril. Relax your fingers and exhale through both nostrils.

2 Close your right nostril with your thumb and inhale in your left nostril to a count of four. Hold both nostrils closed to a count of four. Open your right nostril and exhale to a count of four. Repeat, closing your left nostril. *Repetitions:* Repeat the entire sequence three to four times.

BREATHING EXERCISES

Invigorating Breath

Aim: To ease tension and relax your lower back muscles and hamstrings.

Starting Position: Standing erect.

1 Inhale deeply while extending your arms straight out in front of you, with your palms down (this action fills the lower part of your lungs).

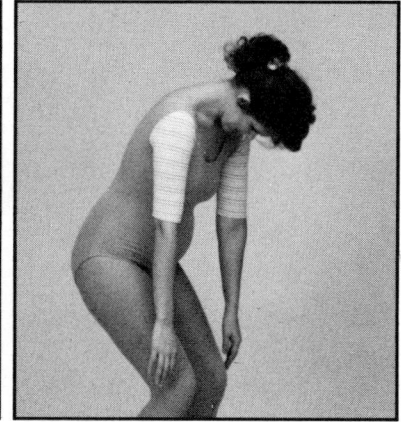

2 Inhale again and extend your arms sideways, with your palms down (this action fills the middle part of your lungs).

3 Inhale as you raise your arms overhead (keeping your arms straight) until your palms touch (this action fills the upper portion of your lungs).

4 Completely relax your body. Exhale through your mouth as you let your upper body fall forward like a limp rag doll, flexing your knees slightly and keeping your fingers as close to the floor as possible.

BREATHING EXERCISES

Yoga Breathing/Stretch

Aim: To relieve upper-back ache, shortness of breath, and indigestion, and to allow practice in breathing correctly while exercising.

Starting Position: Standing erect, arms stretched in front of you, hands locked together, palms facing out.

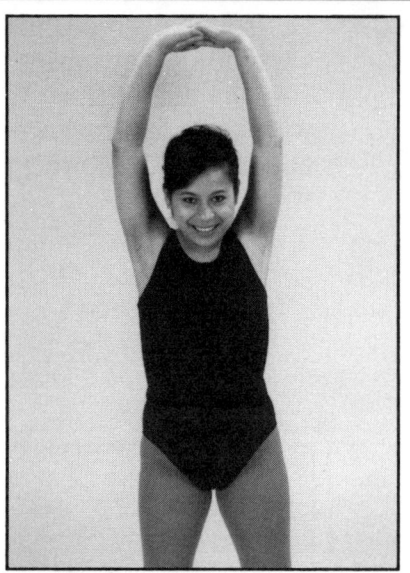

1 Inhale deeply while raising your arms above your head, straight up.

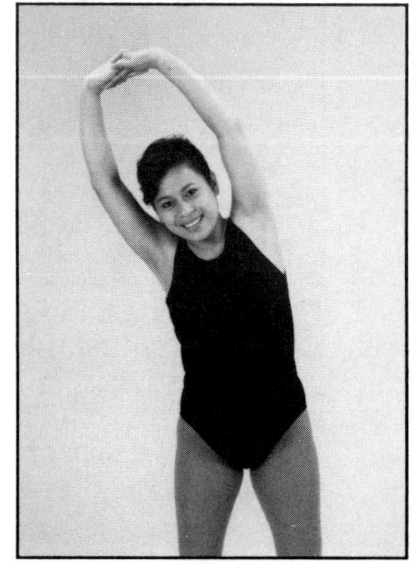

2 Exhale as you bend your upper body to the right. Make sure your knees are slightly bent. Straighten your upper body and return to starting position. Inhale as you raise your arms above your head. Exhale and bend your upper body to the left.
Repetitions: Repeat three to five times on each side.

PRENATAL EXERCISES

Exercise No. 1

1 Begin with a few simple breaths.

⬥Head Arcs

Aim: To loosen up your neck and shoulders.
Starting Position: Tailor sit.

2 Lower your head toward your left shoulder; return to starting position. Lower your head toward your right shoulder; return to starting position.

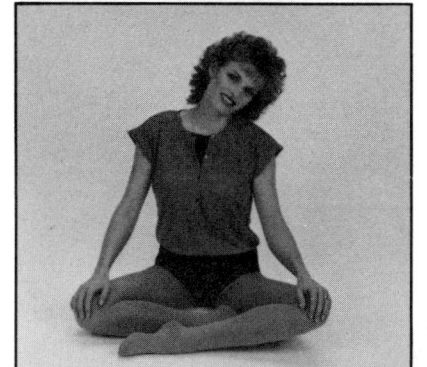

3 Roll your chin to your chest and back up again.

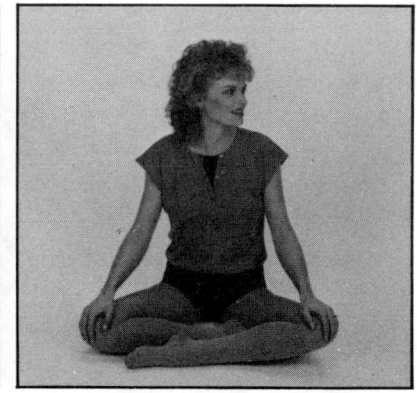

4 Turn your head to look left, then right. *Repetitions:* Repeat three times.

PRENATAL EXERCISES

Exercise No. 2

Face Exercises

Aim: To tighten your facial muscles.

Starting Position: Tailor sit.

1 Smile.

2 Pucker your face, then relax.

Note: Also try exercising your face by chewing gum and forming vowel sounds or words with your mouth.

PRENATAL EXERCISES

Exercise No. 3

1 Raise your left knee to your chest.

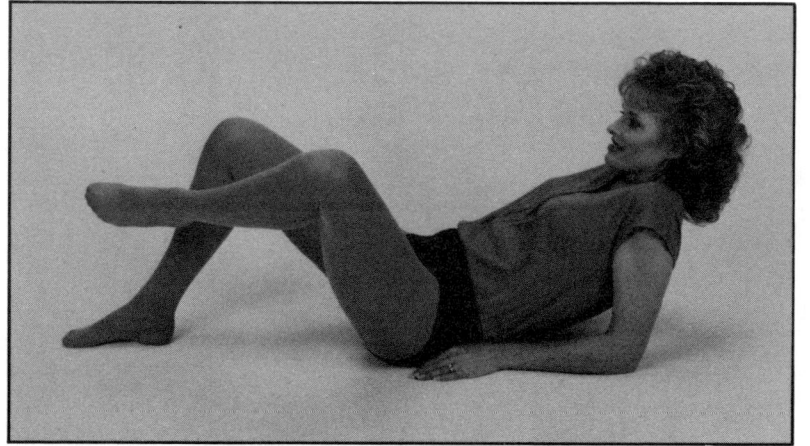

2 With your left knee, trace a large circle directly in front of your body. Rotate your leg ten times to the left, then ten times to the right. Repeat with your right leg. *Repetitions:* Do one set with each leg.

Hip/Knee Rotations

Aim: To promote flexibility in your hip and knee joints.
Starting Position: Hook-lying, resting on your elbows.

PRENATAL EXERCISES

Exercise No. 4

Shoulders

Aim: To loosen up your shoulders and tone your upper arms.

Starting Position: Standing with your feet slightly apart and your arms at your sides; may also be done sitting.

1 *Rotations:* Raise your shoulders to your ears. Pull your shoulders back and downward, then up and forward.

2 With your left shoulder, "draw" three circles forward, then three circles backward. Repeat with your right shoulder. Draw three circles forward with both shoulders, then reverse and draw three circles backward.

1 *Lifts:* Lift your shoulders and roll them forward. With your palms facing out, bring your arms forward until your little fingers touch.

2 Lift your shoulders again and roll them backwards. With your palms still facing out, bring your arms behind your body until you feel the stretch in your shoulders.
Repetitions: Repeat three times.

PRENATAL EXERCISES

Exercise No. 4

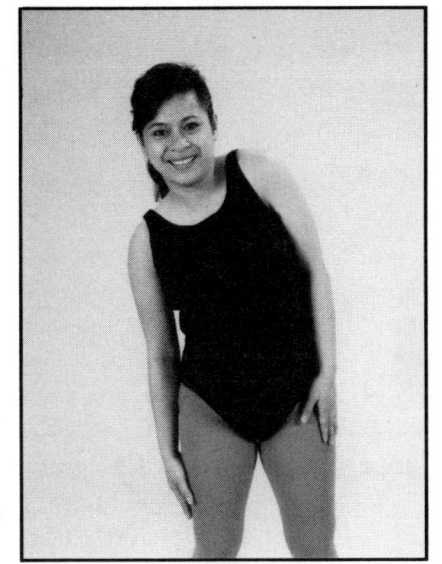

◊ Shoulders

Aim: To loosen up your shoulders and tone your upper arms.

Starting Position: Standing with your feet slightly apart and your arms at your sides; may also be done sitting.

Note: Never drop your head and shoulders to the back.

1 Tuck your pelvis in and pull in your abdominal muscles. Keep them tucked throughout this exercise. Lean your head and upper body to the right. Return to starting position.

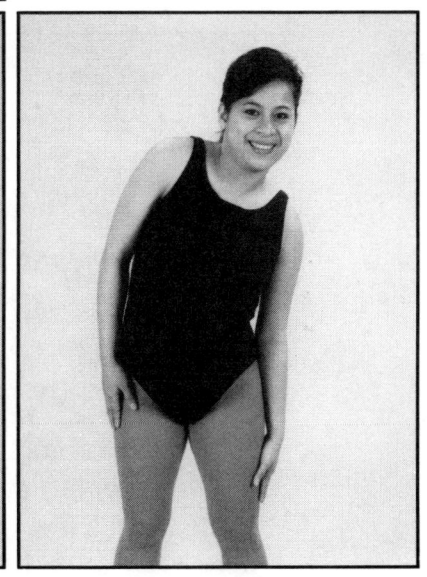

2 Roll both shoulders forward and let your head drop forward slightly. Extend your arms down in front of you with the backs of your hands touching. Return to starting position.

3 Lean your head and upper body to the left. Return to starting position. *Repetitions:* Repeat 3 times, alternating from left to right.

25

PRENATAL EXERCISES

Exercise No. 5

Arms

Aim: To tone and loosen up your arms, wrists, and fingers.

Starting Position: Standing or sitting with your arms straight out in front of you, palms up.

1 *Curls:* Squeeze your hands to form fists.

2 Touch your fists to your shoulders, then straighten your arms.
Repetitions: Repeat three to five times.

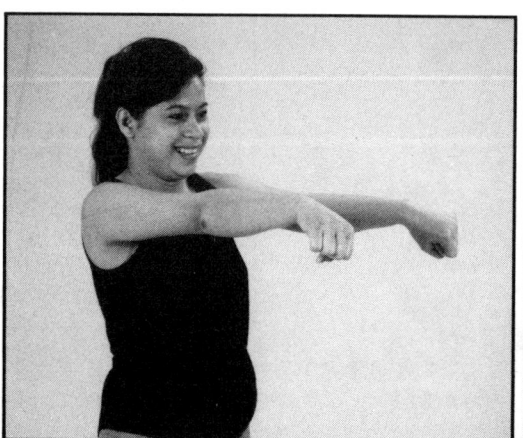

Wrist Rotations: Make fists and circle them a few times to the left, then a few times to the right.

Finger Flowers: Make fists, then slowly open your fingers like a flower opening.

PRENATAL EXERCISES

Exercise No. 6

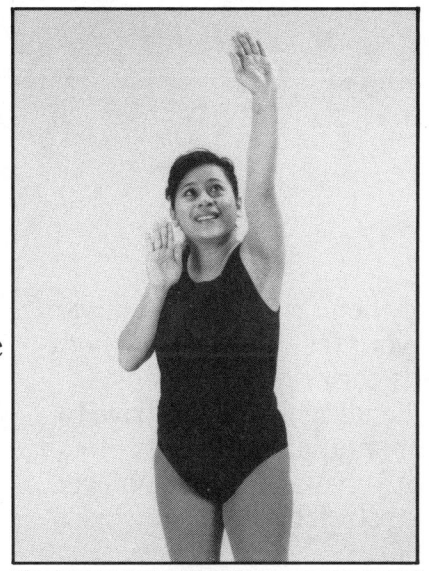

1 Press the palm of your left hand toward the ceiling, stretching the entire left side of your body until your left heel rises slightly off the floor. *Repetitions:* Repeat on your right side, then on your left side, then again on your right side.

Raggedy Ann

Aim: To loosen up and relax your body, particularly your neck, shoulders, and legs. This exercise can be done at any time during the exercise routine.

Starting Position: Standing, with your feet shoulder-width apart, your knees bent, and your toes and knees aligned.

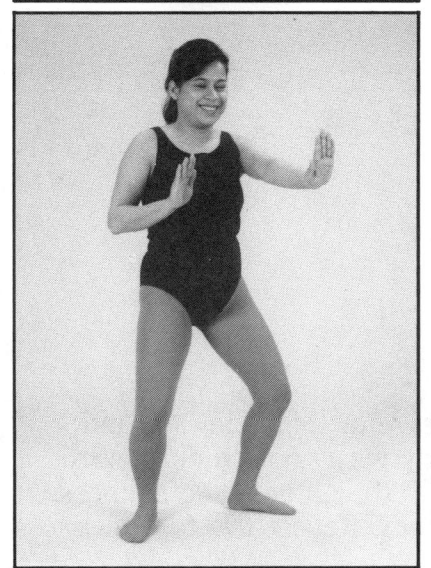

2 With your knees slightly bent, round your shoulders and raise your arms to shoulder level. Alternately press forward with your left hand, then with your right hand, as if pushing an object away.

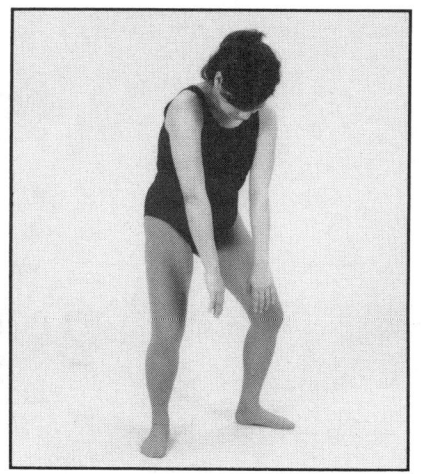

3 Keeping your hips in line with your shoulders, drop your head forward with your chin to your chest. Round your shoulders forward, bend your knees, and roll up to starting position. *Repetitions:* Repeat the entire exercise one to three times.

27

PRENATAL EXERCISES

Exercise No. 7

Pliés ◊

Aim: To strengthen your lower back and legs.

Starting Position: Standing erect with your feet shoulder-width apart, your pelvis tucked, your abdominal muscles pulled in, your knees bent, and your toes and knees aligned.

1 Slowly bend your knees outward over your feet. Lower your body as far as is comfortably possible without bending forward. Strive to keep your shoulders aligned with your hips. When you have achieved maximum stretch, push your heels to the floor.

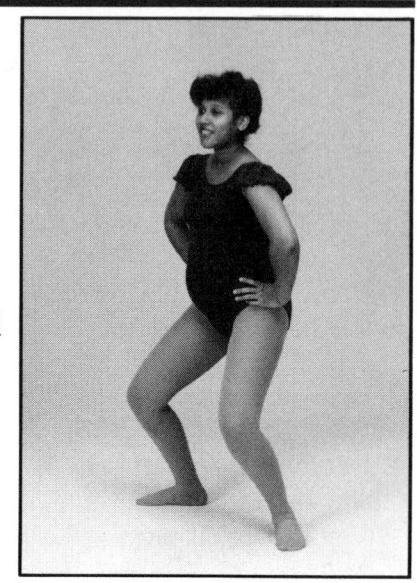

2 Press your thighs inward and slowly push your trunk upward, gradually straightening your knees.
Repetitions: Repeat five to fifteen times.

PRENATAL EXERCISES

Exercise No. 8

Start-Up Stretch

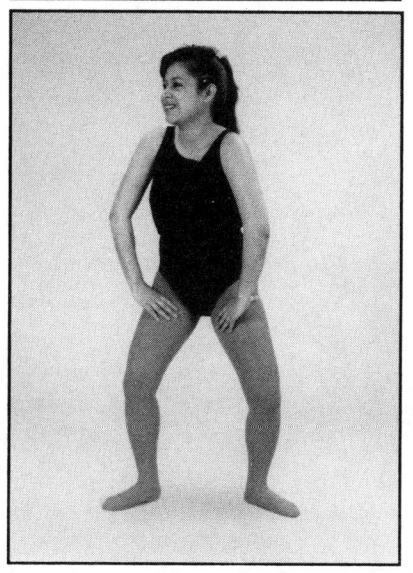

1 Place your hands on your upper anterior thighs and press your right shoulder toward your left shoulder.

2 Repeat, pressing your left shoulder toward your right shoulder.
Repetitions: Repeat ten times to each side.

Aim: To loosen up your arms and shoulders and stretch your lower back.

Starting Position: Standing, with your feet shoulder-width apart, your knees bent, and your toes and knees aligned.

PRENATAL EXERCISES

Exercise Nos. 9 and 10

Butterfly Rock

Aim: To stretch your inner thighs and help prepare you for delivery.

Starting Position: Butterfly sit.

Butterfly Press

Rock: Place your hands on your ankles. Keeping your back straight, rock from side to side three to five times.

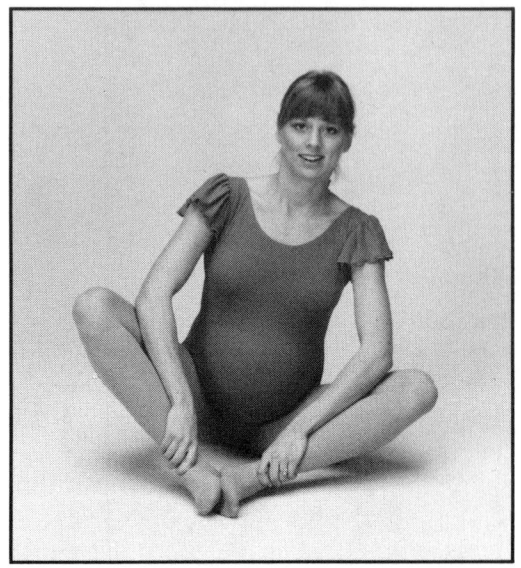

Press: Put your hands on the floor by your hips for support. Keeping your back straight, press your knees slowly to the floor, then return to starting position.
Repetitions: Repeat three to five times.

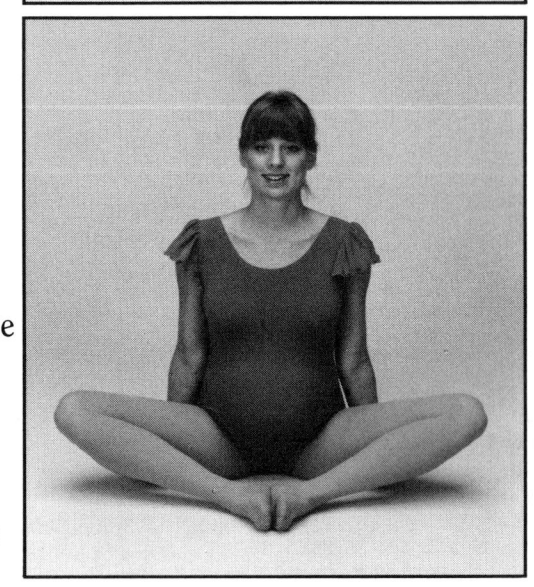

Note: As you gain flexibility, bring your feet closer toward your body for more stretching.

PRENATAL EXERCISES

Exercise No. 11

Leg Raisers

Aim: To strengthen your abdominal and buttock muscles, lower back, and legs.

Starting Position: Hook-lying, resting on your elbows.

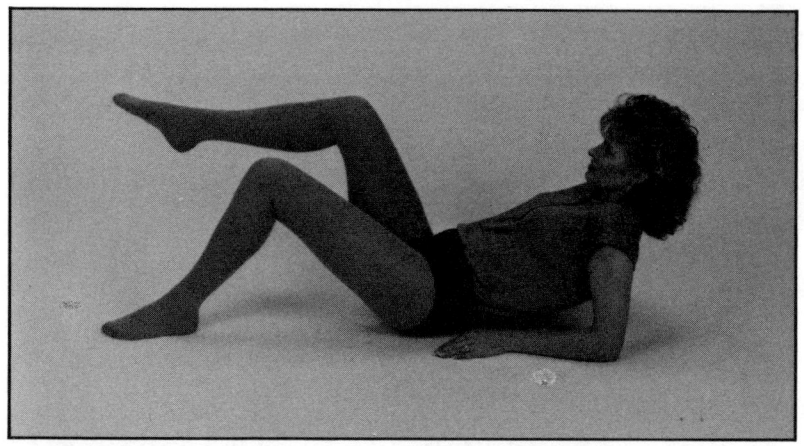

1 Draw your right leg to your chest. Extend your right leg to the ceiling, pointing your toes as you do so. Press your lower back to the floor.

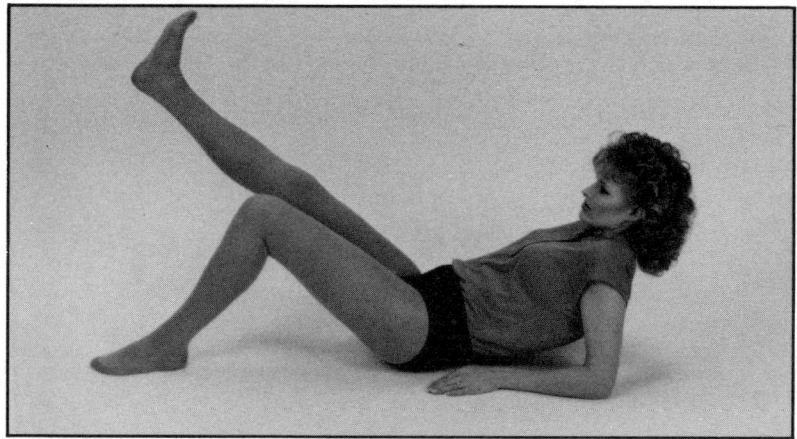

2 Flex your right foot and lower your leg slowly to the floor. *Repetitions:* Repeat three to five times with each leg.

PRENATAL EXERCISES

Exercise No. 12

Pelvic Rock
(on your back)

Aim: To soothe your lower back, strengthen your abdominal muscles, and prepare you for delivery.

Starting Position: Hook-lying.

1 Press your lower back to the floor. Hold this position for a few seconds, then relax. *Repetitions:* Repeat five times *slowly*.

Note: After your fourth month of pregnancy, do the pelvic rock on all fours.

PRENATAL EXERCISES

Exercise No. 13

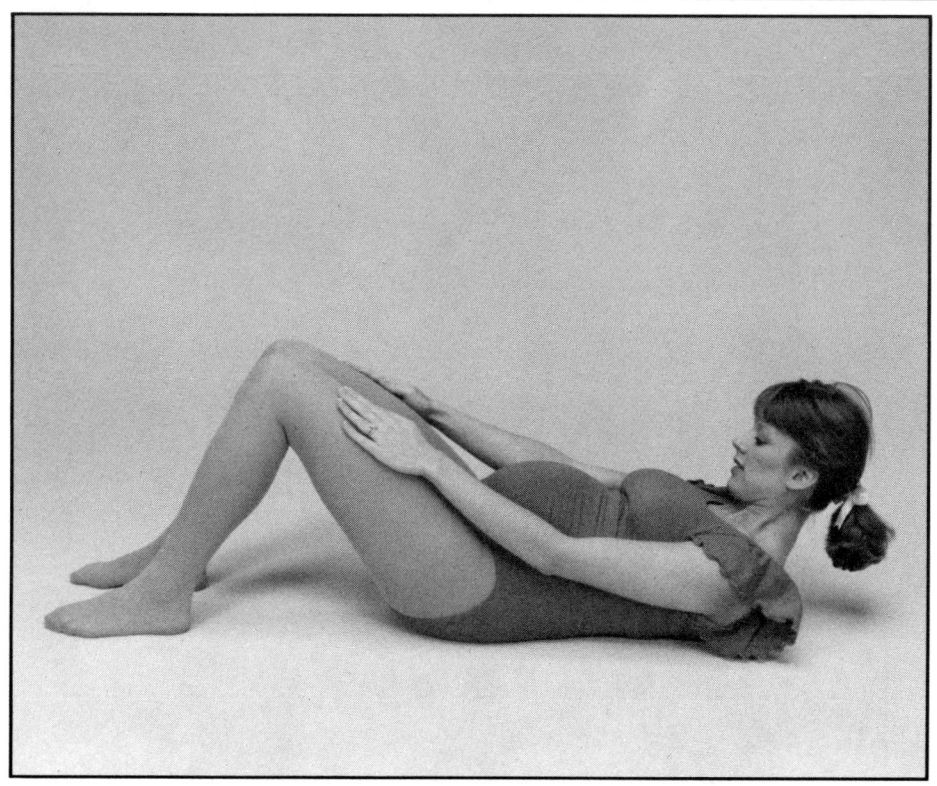

Curl-Ups

Aim: To strengthen your abdominal muscles and lower back.

Starting Position: Hook-lying.

1 Holding your chin to your chest, curl up slowly just far enough for your shoulder blades to come off the floor. Hold your head and neck tightly in a fixed position for a few seconds, then lower your back to the floor. *Repetitions:* Repeat three to five times.

Note: After your fourth month of pregnancy, limit the time spent on this exercise to three minutes or less. If you feel light-headed, omit the exercise completely or do Sit-Backs (Exercise No. 34, p. 58).

PRENATAL EXERCISES

Exercise No. 13

Oblique Curl-Ups

Aim: To strengthen your oblique abdominal muscles.

Starting Position: Hook-lying.

Curl up slowly, lifting your right shoulder toward your left side; stretch your arms to the left side. Repeat to the right side. *Repetitions:* Repeat three to five times on each side, alternating.

Note: After your fourth month of pregnancy, limit the time spent on this exercise to three minutes or less. If you feel light-headed, omit the exercise completely or do Sit-Backs (Exercise No. 34, p. 58).

PRENATAL EXERCISES

Exercise No. 14

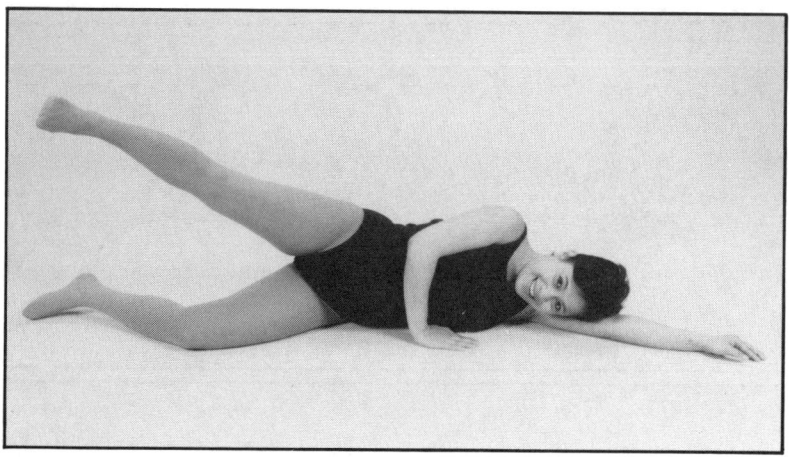

1 Raise your right leg to a comfortable height and hold it there. Circle your foot to the left, then to the right.

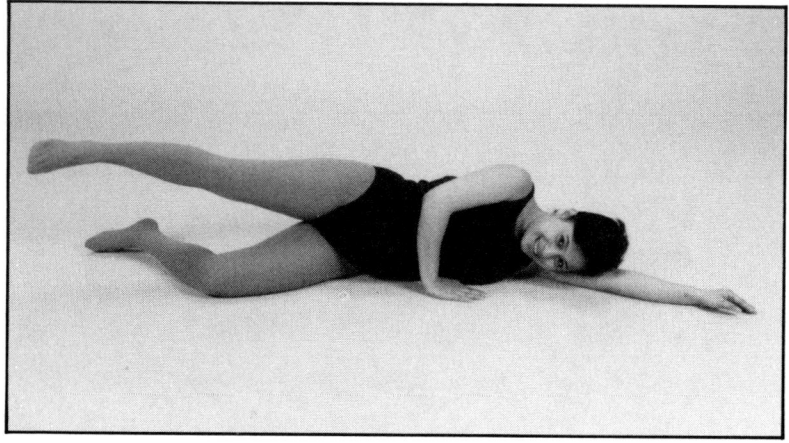

2 Lower your leg to hip level, hold it there, and circle your foot again.

Raise and Roll

Aim: To strengthen your abdominal muscles, quadriceps, ankles, buttocks, and outer thigh muscles.

Starting Position: Lying on your left side with your left knee bent, your right leg extended, and resting your head on your left arm.

PRENATAL EXERCISES

Exercise No. 14

3 Lower your leg nearly to the floor and circle your foot. *Repetitions:* Repeat steps 1 through 3 three to five times.

4 With your left knee still bent, extend your right leg in front of you and touch knees. With your foot flexed, raise your right leg to hip level, then lower it. *Repetitions:* Repeat three to five times, then roll to your right side and repeat the entire exercise with your left leg.

PRENATAL EXERCISES

Exercise No. 15

Cheek-to-Cheek

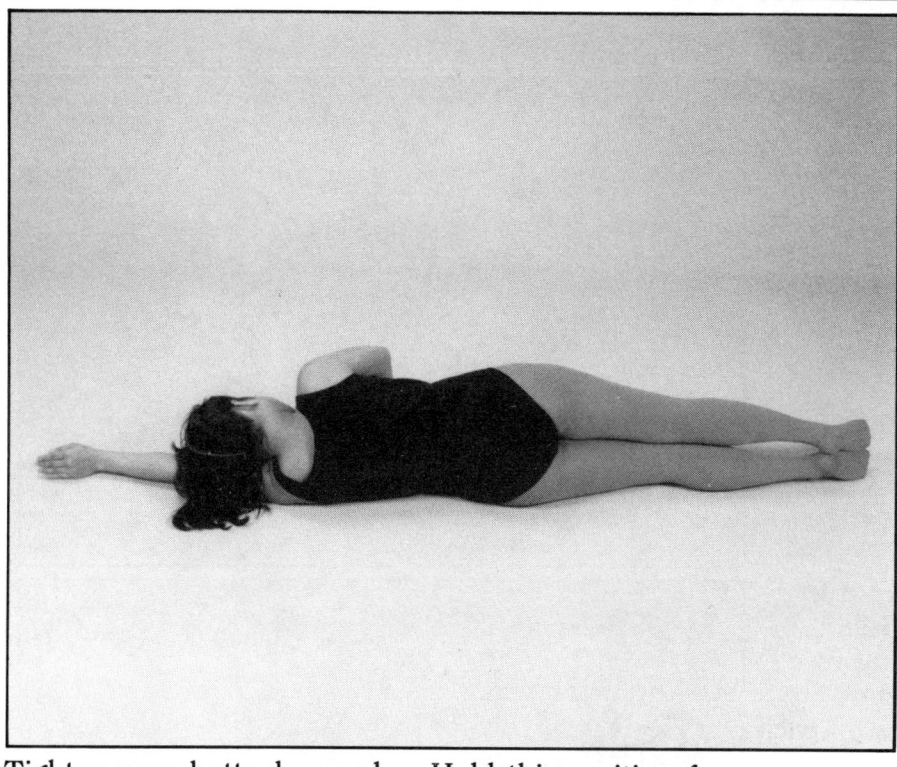

Tighten your buttock muscles. Hold this position for fifteen seconds, and then release. *Repetitions:* Repeat three to five times.

Aim: To tone your buttock muscles.

Starting Position: Lying on your left side, with right leg directly on top of your left leg and knees slightly bent. Rest your head on your left arm and use your right arm to steady your body.

PRENATAL EXERCISES

Exercise No. 16

Hip Rock

Aim: To trim your waistline and tone your arms and pectoral muscles.

Starting Position: All fours.

1 Inhale as you rock your left hip to the side and look around your left arm.

2 Exhale and return to the all-fours position then repeat, rocking your right hip. *Repetitions:* Repeat three times on each side, alternating sides.

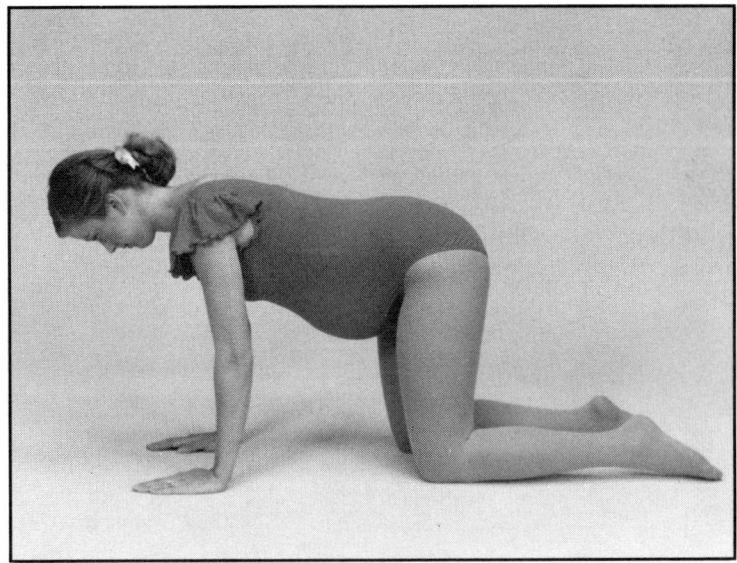

PRENATAL EXERCISES

Exercise No. 17

Pelvic Rock
(on all fours)

Aim: To soothe your back muscles, strengthen your arms, lower back and abdominal muscles, and prepare you for delivery.

Starting Position: All fours.

Raise your back slightly and hold the position for a few seconds. Return to starting position. *Repetitions:* Repeat three to five times, very slowly.

Note: To avoid any strain on the lower back, never let your back sag during this exercise and keep your elbows, head, and knees still.

PRENATAL EXERCISES

Exercise No. 18

Leg Extenders

Aim: To strengthen your lower back, abdominal muscles, pectoral muscles, hamstrings, and buttock muscles.

Starting Position: All fours.

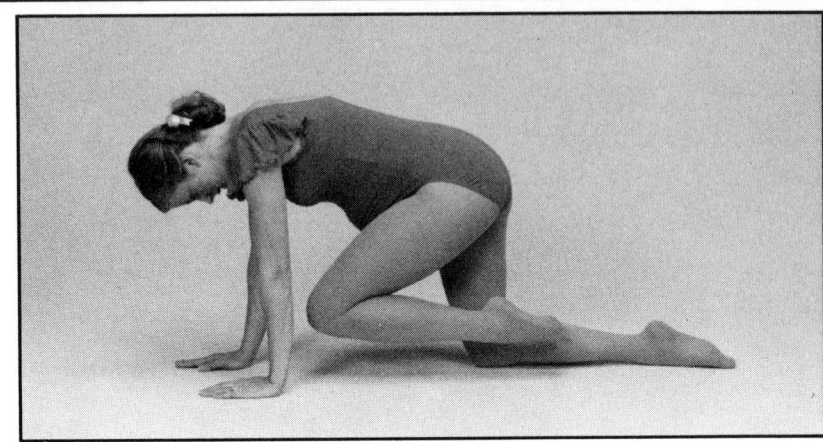

1 Bring your left knee forward, toward your chin.

2 Slowly extend your leg back, keeping your knee slightly bent. *Repetitions:* Repeat three times with your left leg, then three times with your right leg. Do a pelvic rock (raise your back slightly), then return to all-fours position.

Note: To avoid any strain on the lower back, never let your back sag during this exercise and keep your elbows, head, and knees still.

PRENATAL EXERCISES

Exercise No. 19

1 Bring your right knee toward your chest.

2 Slowly extend your right leg back to starting position.
Repetitions: Repeat three to five times with right leg, then roll over to right side and repeat three to five times with left leg.

Leg Extenders
(variation)

Aim: To strengthen your lower back, abdominal muscles, pectoral muscles, hamstrings, and buttock muscles.

Starting Position: Lying on your left side with your left knee slightly bent, your right leg extended, and resting your head on your left arm.

PRENATAL EXERCISES

Exercise No. 20

Open Pelvic Rock

Aim: To strengthen your abdominal muscles, pelvic floor muscles, inner and outer thigh muscles, shoulders, and neck; and to help prepare you for delivery.

Starting Position: Lying on your back, with the soles of your feet together in the butterfly position.

Notes: After your fourth month of pregnancy, you may switch to the Sitting Pelvic Stretch exercise (No. 33, p. 57).

Breathe in, then out as you do the exercise; do not hold your breath. In preparation for delivery, practice relaxing your face during the exercise; but never practice actual pushing.

1 Bring your feet as close to your body as possible, keeping your head up and your shoulder blades off the floor. Press your heels together.

2 Holding your ankles with your hands, pull your ankles toward your chin. At the same time, move your knees outward *only* until you feel a stretch in your inner thigh muscles.

Repetitions: Repeat three to five times.

PRENATAL EXERCISES

Exercise No. 21

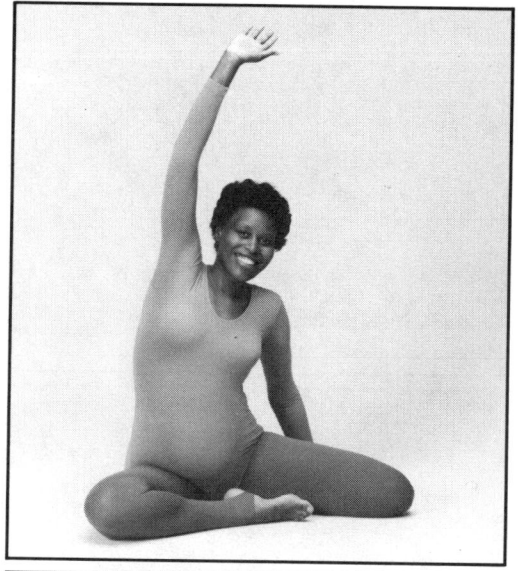

1 Bend to the left and press your right palm slowly toward the ceiling, steadying yourself with your left arm if necessary.

2 Return to starting position, then bend to the right and press your left palm toward the ceiling.
Repetitions: Repeat five times slowly on each side, alternating sides.

◊ Stretch and Press

Aim: To tone your arms, waist, and lower back.

Starting Position: Side sit or tailor sit.

Notes: If you have bad knees, extend your back leg to a straight position for a modified side sit.

Breathe in and out normally as you do the exercise.

To do this exercise in water, stand and hold onto the side of the pool.

PRENATAL EXERCISES

Exercise No. 22

Leg and Foot Toner

Aim: To stretch and tone your leg and foot muscles and to improve your circulation; done daily, it can help to prevent leg and foot cramps.

Starting Position: Pike sit with your arms behind you and your palms flat on the floor.

To do this exercise in water, stand and hold onto the side of the pool.

1 *Point:* Tighten your leg and buttock muscles. Point your toes, stretch, then relax. *Repetitions:* Repeat five times, then shake out your legs.

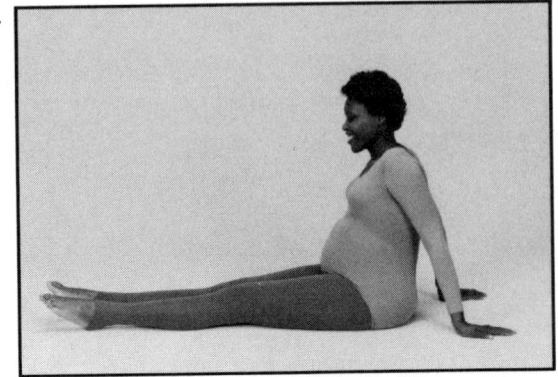

2 *Flex:* Point your toes toward the ceiling. Hold the position as you tighten your leg and buttock muscles, then relax. *Repetitions:* Repeat five times, then shake out your legs.

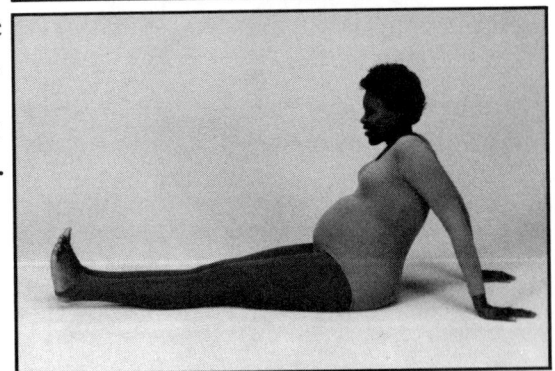

3 *Circle:* Keeping your feet flat on the floor, bend your knees. Lean back and rest on your forearms. Rest your right leg on your left knee and circle your right foot five times to the left, then five times to the right, flexing your foot and pointing your toes as you do so. *Repetitions:* Repeat with your left foot.

PRENATAL EXERCISES

Exercise No. 23

1 Lean forward, placing your hands on the floor in front of your legs in a trapezoid ⏢ form.

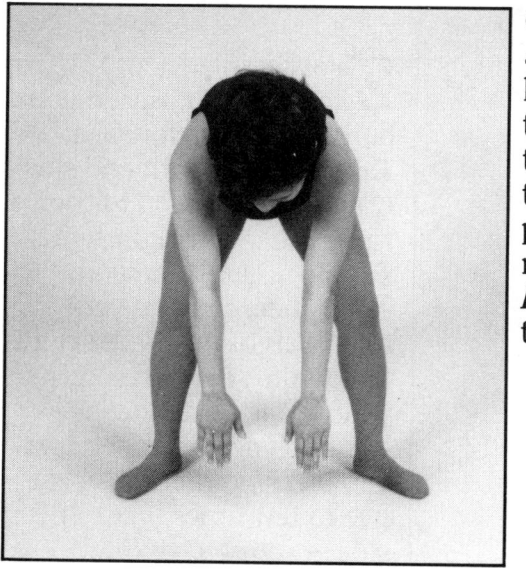

2 Straighten your legs as much as you can, keeping your feet flat on the floor and your hands touching or reaching toward the floor. Hold this position, then relax and return to starting position.
Repetitions: Repeat five times.

Squats

Aim: To strengthen your inner and outer thigh muscles and to prepare you for pushing during delivery.

Starting Position: Standing with your legs apart and your hands on your hips, with feet pointed out and your knees bent so that your hips are at knee level.

Notes: Squat no deeper than stool height. Going lower may hurt your knees.

Also, never practice actual pushing while doing the exercise.

45

PRENATAL EXERCISES

Exercise No. 24

Breathe and Lunge

Aim: To strengthen your hips and leg muscles.

Starting Position: Standing with your hands on your hips and your feet two to three feet apart.

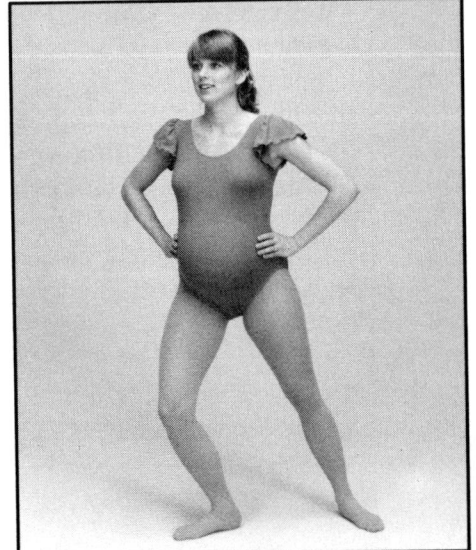

1 Take a deep breath and slowly step forward and to the left with your left foot. Exhale as you bend your left knee, shifting your body weight onto your left foot while striving to keep your right leg extended. Lunge as deeply as comfort allows.

2 Pause, inhale, and return to starting position with both feet facing forward. Take a deep breath and slowly step forward and to the right with your right foot. Exhale as you bend your right knee, shifting your body weight onto your right foot while striving to keep your left leg extended. Lunge as deeply as comfort allows. *Repetitions:* Repeat five to ten times on each side.

Note: You may add the Yoga Breathing Stretch (see page 20) here once you learn it.

PRENATAL EXERCISES

Exercise No. 25

Scissors: Hold your arms out, straight in front of your body, with your palms down. Move your arms in a scissors motion, alternating right over left arm and left over right arm. *Repetitions:* Repeat the entire exercise with your palms up ten times and with your palms down ten times.

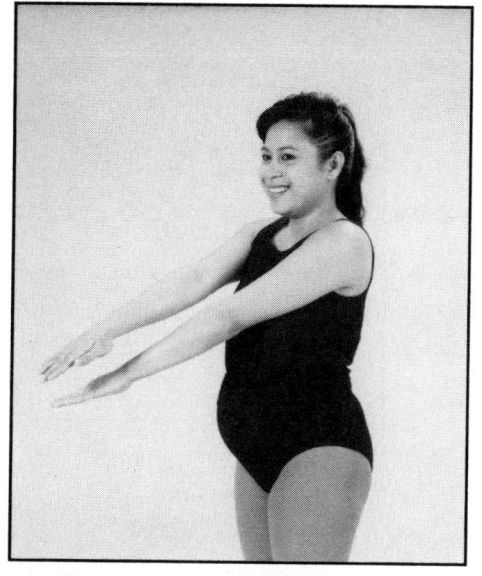

◊ Arm Series

Aim: To strengthen your upper and lower arms, wrists, and pectoral muscles.

Starting Position: Standing, with your feet shoulder-width apart and your arms in cross position.

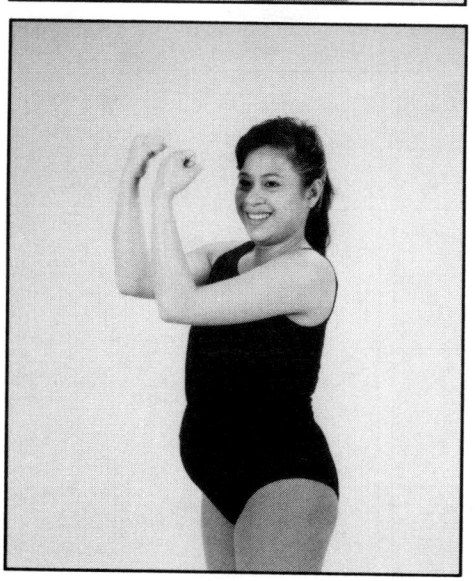

Elbows Together: Bend your arms at the elbows. Tightening your arms, make fists, and bring your forearms together in front of your body. Press your arms open to cross position. *Repetitions:* Repeat five to ten times.

47

PRENATAL EXERCISES

Exercise No. 26

Arm Series 💧

Aim: To strengthen your upper and lower arms, wrists, and pectoral muscles.

Starting Position: Standing with your feet shoulders'-width apart and your arms in cross position.

Push Backs: Turn your palms away from your back and gently press up. *Repetitions:* Repeat five times.

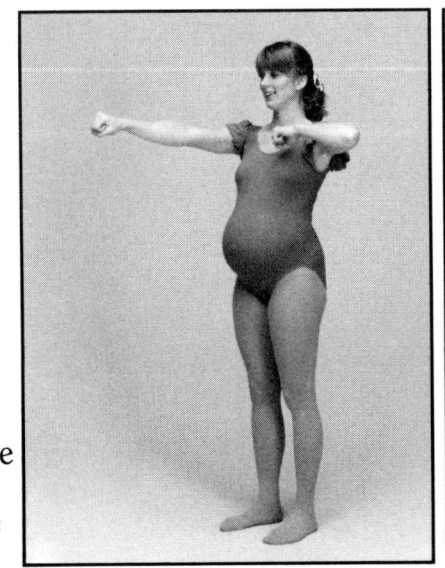

1 *Arm Punches:* Make fists. Punch forward five times, alternating arms. Punch over your head five times, alternating arms.

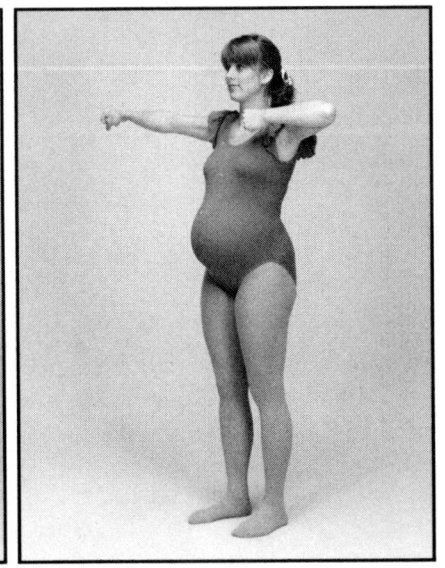

2 Punch out to your sides five times, alternating arms.

PRENATAL EXERCISES

Exercise No. 26

Arm Circles: With your palms up, move your arms forward to make five small circles, then five large circles. *Repetitions:* Repeat, moving your arms backward, then repeat with your palms down.

Wrist Flexors: Moving only your wrists, point your fingertips toward the floor. *Repetitions:* Repeat five times.

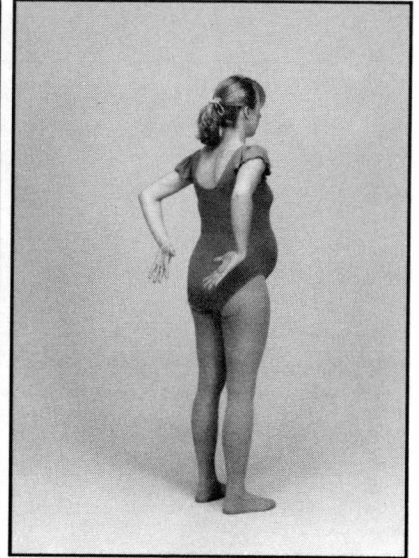

Scarecrow: With palms down, spread your fingers. Bend your arms at your elbows and swing your palms in front of your body. Return to starting position. *Repetitions:* Repeat five times.

Back Sweeper: With palms down, spread your fingers. Bend your arms at the elbows and try to touch your fingertips behind your back. Return to starting position. *Repetitions:* Repeat five times.

PRENATAL EXERCISES

Exercise No. 26

Arm Series

Aim: To strengthen your upper and lower arms, wrists, and pectoral muscles.

Starting Position: Standing with your feet shoulder-width apart and your arms in cross position.

1 *Elbow Flex:* With your palms up, make fists.

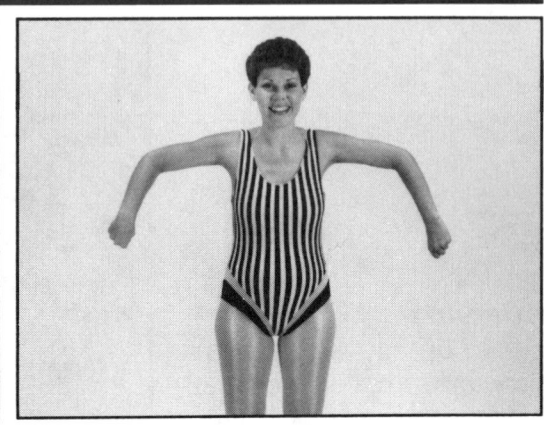

2 Bend your elbows until your fists touch your shoulders, then circle your forearms downward and outward until extended.

3 Turn your fists toward the ceiling.

4 Bend your elbows and touch your fists to your shoulders, then return to starting position. *Repetitions:* Repeat entire exercise five times.

PRENATAL EXERCISES

Exercise No. 28

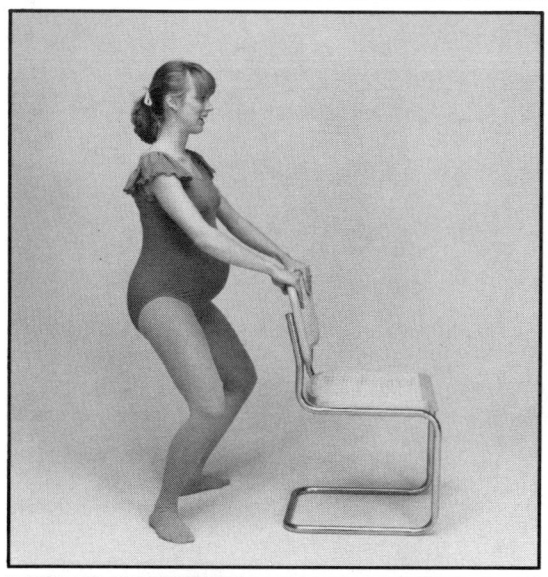

1. Slowly bend both knees, pressing your feet into the floor as if to sit on a stool. Hold the position for five seconds.

❧ Standing Thigh Stretch

Aim: To tone your entire body, especially your legs and inner thighs.

Starting Position: Standing with your legs apart and your toes pointing out.

2. Slowly stretch up, keeping your legs tight and your feet flat on the floor as you return to starting position. *Repetitions:* Repeat five times.

Note: Balance against a chair, wall, or bar for support if balance is a problem.

51

PRENATAL EXERCISES

Exercise No. 28

Wall Push-Ups

Aim: To strengthen your shoulders and pectoral muscles, and to develop the arm muscles that you use in pushing during delivery.

Starting Position: Standing an arm's length or further from a wall, with your legs comfortably apart.

1 Place your hands on the wall, with your fingertips pointed in and your elbows parallel to the floor.

2 Keep your feet flat on the floor, inhale as you slowly lean toward the wall. Exhale as you slowly push away from the wall. *Repetitions:* Do ten or twenty push-ups.

PRENATAL EXERCISES

Exercise No. 29

◊ Calf Stretch

Aim: To stretch your calves in preparation for the walking portion of the exercise routine.

Starting Position: Standing an arm's length from the wall, with your palms flat against the wall, toes pointed forward, and hips pressed forward.

Step forward with your right foot, bending your right knee, and stretch your left leg behind you (keep both heels on the floor). Keeping your lower back flat, hold a comfortable stretch for fifteen seconds. Do not bounce. Return to starting position. *Repetitions:* Repeat with your left foot forward.

PRENATAL EXERCISES

Exercise No. 30

Skier's Sit 💧

Aim: To strengthen your legs, abdominal muscles, and lower back.

Starting Position: Standing with your back against a wall.

1 Bend your knees and slide your upper body down. "Sit" with your thighs at a right angle to the wall, as if you were sitting on a stool. Press the small of your back firmly against the wall. (This is a great time to practice kegels. See page 6.) Hold this position for twenty to forty-five seconds.

2 Lean forward and place your hands on your knees, then slowly straighten your back. Straighten your knees slowly and return to a standing position.

Walking 💧

Aim: To strengthen your cardiovascular system and your legs.

Walk briskly. Strive for fifteen to twenty minutes of walking with your heart rate between fifty and seventy percent of your maximum target heart rate. (See pages 8 to 10 for information about the cardiovascular system and target heart rate.)

PRENATAL EXERCISES

Exercise No. 31

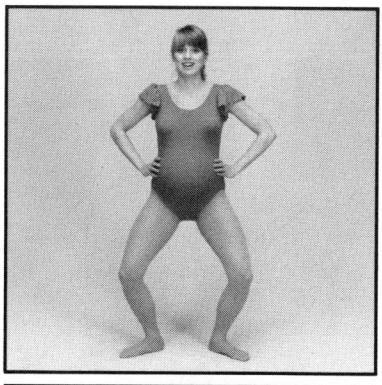

1 *Side-to-side sway:* Sway from side to side, keeping your hips and shoulders in vertical alignment. *Repetitions:* Repeat five times.

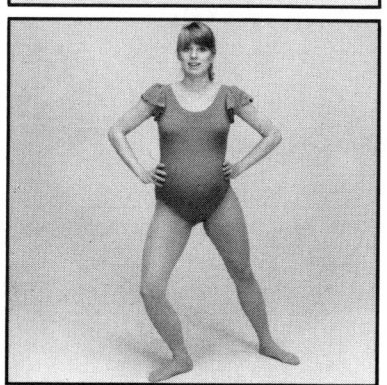

2 *Stride Sway:* Keeping your feet shoulder-width apart, take one step forward with your right foot. Sway forward and back, keeping your heels on the floor. *Repetitions:* Repeat ten times with your right foot and ten with your left.

3 *Elbow-hip sway:* Place your hands on your shoulders and lower your right elbow to your right hip, then return to upright position. Lower your left elbow to your left hip, then return to starting position. *Repetitions:* Repeat ten times, alternating sides.

◊ Plié Series

Aim: To tone your legs, waist, buttock muscles, and lower back.

Starting Position: Standing erect with your feet shoulder-width apart, your pelvis tucked, your abdominal muscles pulled in, your knees bent, and your toes and knees aligned.

Note: To do this exercise in water, stand in shallow water.
Starting Position: Standing erect with your feet shoulder-width apart, your pelvis tucked, your abdominal muscles pulled in, your knees bent, and your toes and knees aligned.

PRENATAL EXERCISES

Exercise No. 32

Backache Relievers

Aim: To stretch your lower back, inner thighs, and pectoral muscles.

Starting Position: Tailor sit.

1 Round your shoulders until you feel a good stretch across the shoulder blades. Do not initiate the move forward from the head—you could strain your lower back. Keep your head up and your lower back flat.

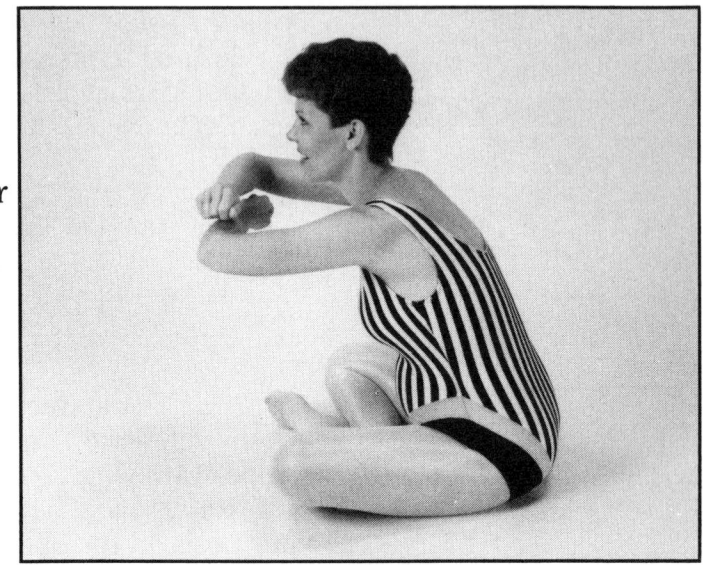

2 Draw your elbows back, keeping your arms parallel to the floor and pinching your shoulder blades together.

PRENATAL EXERCISES

Exercise No. 33

Sitting Pelvic Stretch

Aim: To strengthen your pelvic floor and inner thighs.

Starting Position: Butterfly sit, holding your ankles.

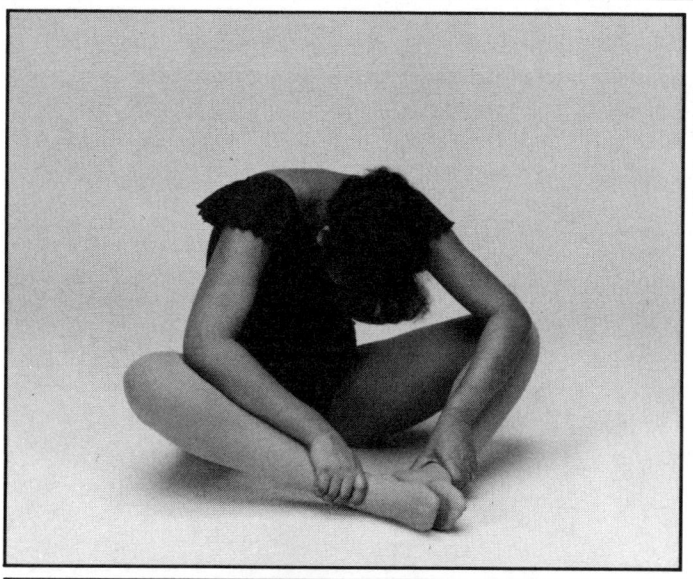

1 Inhale, then exhale as you pull in your abdomen, lower your head as close to your feet as you can, and use your elbows to press your knees to the floor.

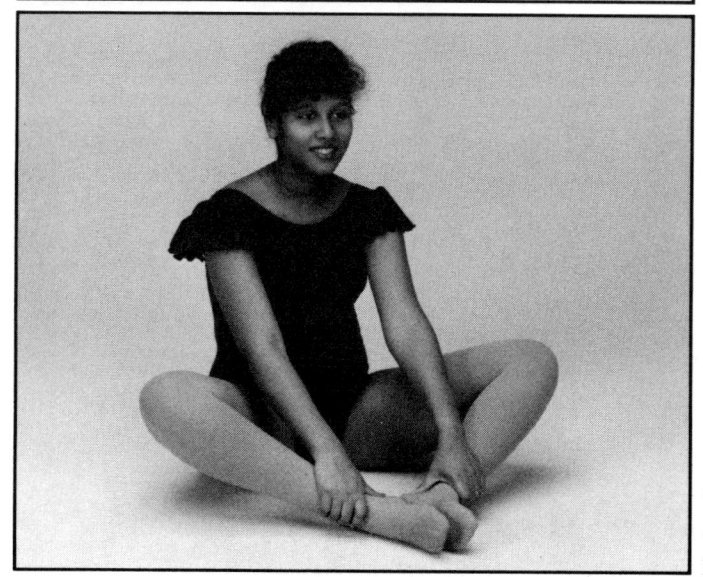

2 Return to starting position. *Repetitions:* Repeat five times.

PRENATAL EXERCISES

Exercise No. 34

Sit-Backs

Aim: To strengthen your abdominal muscles.

Starting Position: Pike sit; bend your knees to your chest, with your hands holding behind your knees.

1 Holding behind your knees, tuck your chin into your chest, and slowly straighten your arms as far as you can. Hold for five counts.

2 Slowly pull with your arms and return to the starting position.
Repetitions: Repeat the entire exercise five to ten times.

Note: In this exercise, safety is maintained by holding behind your knees.

PRENATAL EXERCISES
Exercise No. 35

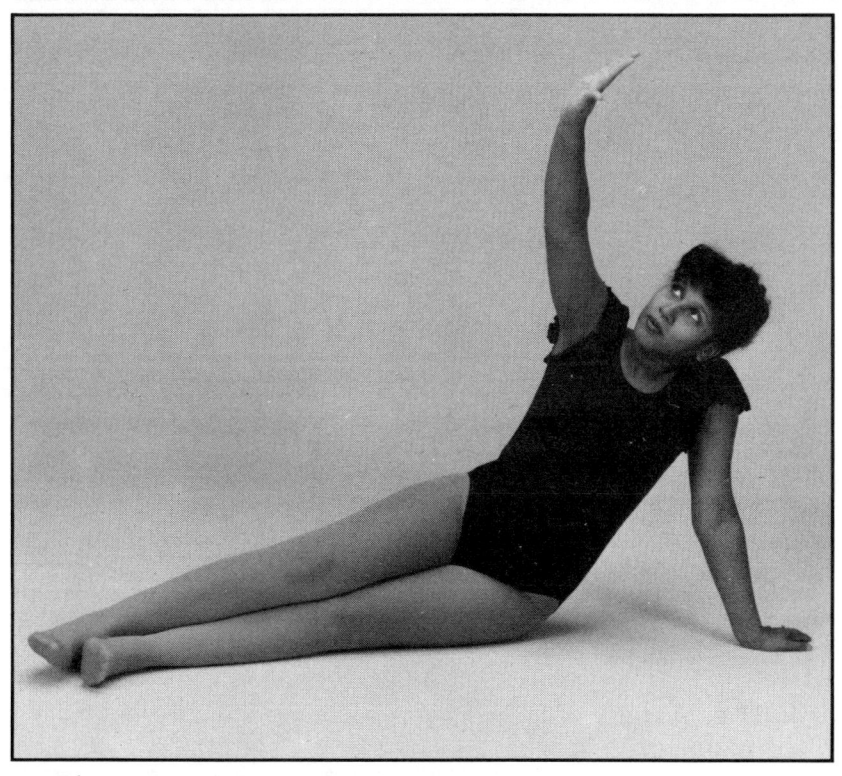

Thigh Roll

Aim: To tone your waistline, hips, outer thighs, and buttock muscles.

Starting Position: Pike sit.

1 Place your left hand to your side to support your weight. Keeping your left hip on the floor, roll to the left, slightly raising your right hip off the floor as you do so. Press your right palm toward the ceiling as you bend to the left. *Repetitions:* Repeat three to five times on each side, alternating sides, rolling slowly.

PRENATAL EXERCISES

Exercise No. 36

Lateral Straddle Stretch

Aim: To strengthen abdominals, hip flexors, and stretch lower back and hamstrings.

Starting Position: Straddle sit, with your toes pointed comfortably and your arms in cross position.

1. Bend right leg in and bring left arm forward to the inside of your left leg. Bring your right arm over your head and bend to the left. Repeat five times to the left.

2. Bend forward at the center of your body, holding your chest as close to the floor as possible, and return to straddle sit.

3. Bend left leg in and bring right arm forward to the inside of your right leg. Bring your left arm over your head and bend to the right. Repeat five times to the right. Extend your arms in front of you and bend forward at the center of your body, holding your chest as close to the floor as possible and return to straddle sit. *Repetitions:* Repeat the entire exercise once (bending to the right and left five times each).

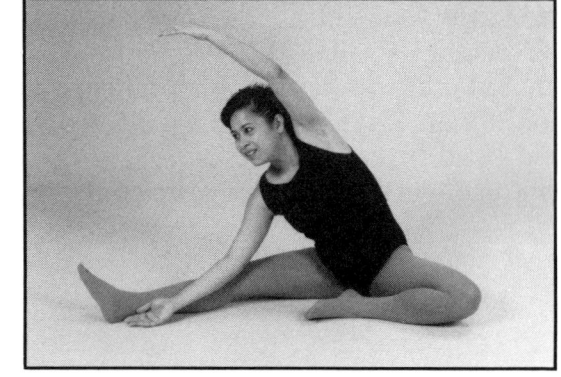

PRENATAL EXERCISES

Exercise No. 37

Hamstring Straddle Stretch

1 Bend right leg in, lean left from your hip and stretch as far forward as you can, looking over your foot. Repeat five times to the left.

2 Bend forward at the center of your body, holding your chest as close to the floor as possible, and return to straddle sit.

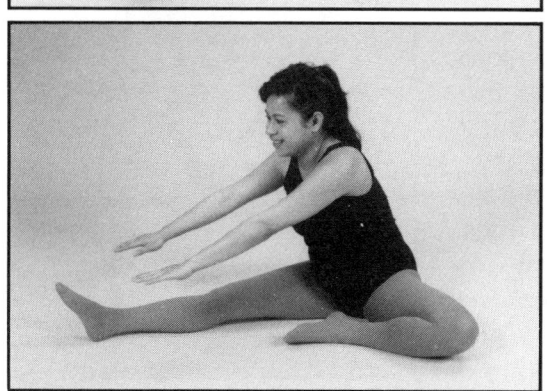

3 Bend left leg in, lean right from your hip and stretch as far forward as you can, looking over your foot. Repeat five times to the right. Bend forward at the center of your body, holding your chest as close to the floor as possible, and return to straddle sit. *Repetitions:* Repeat the entire exercise once (leaning to the left and right five times each).

Aim: To strengthen abdominals, hip flexors, and stretch hamstrings, gluteus, and lower back.

Starting Position: Straddle sit with your toes pointed comfortably and your arms at your sides.

PRENATAL EXERCISES

Exercise No. 38

Shoulder Turns

Aim: To strengthen the oblique muscles, stretch your hips and outer thigh muscles.

Starting Position: Tailor sit.

1 Pick up your left foot and place it outside your right thigh.

2 With your arms in a cross position, inhale, and exhale as you turn to the left. Place your left arm behind you for support, hug your left leg with your right arm, and look over your left shoulder. Hold the position for five seconds, repeat three times slowly, and return to starting position.

3 Pick up your right foot and place it outside your left thigh. With your arms in a cross position, inhale, and exhale as you turn to the right. Place your right arm behind you for support, hug your right leg with your left arm, and look over your right shoulder. Hold the position for five seconds. Repeat three times slowly and return to starting position. *Repetitions:* Repeat the entire exercise once (three times to each side).

PRENATAL EXERCISES

Exercise No. 39

Baby-Go-Round

Aim: To relax your neck, shoulders, and back, and to soothe your ribs.

Starting Position: Tailor sit.

1 Bend your body, head, and shoulders to the right, forward, and to the left in one continuous circular motion. Reverse the circle to the left. *Repetitions:* Alternating directions, do two circles in each direction.

Note: Circle slowly, and never bend backward.

PRENATAL EXERCISES
Exercise No. 40

V-Stretch

Aim: To tone and strengthen your abdominal muscles, legs, feet, and especially your inner thighs.

Starting Position: Back tuck.

1 Open your knees wide, place your toes together, and slide your hands down to your ankles.

2 Pull your feet close to your body, then slowly straighten your legs out to a V position. Hold the position for a few seconds. Do not bounce.

3 Keeping your knees open wide, bring your toes back together, then return to starting position.
Repetitions: Repeat five times.

Note: After your fourth month of pregnancy, be sure to limit the time spent on this exercise to three minutes or less. If you become lightheaded or uncomfortable, try a variation of this exercise.

PRENATAL EXERCISES

Exercise No. 40

V-Stretch

Aim: To tone and strengthen your abdominal muscles, legs, feet, and especially your inner thighs.

Starting Position: Butterfly sit.

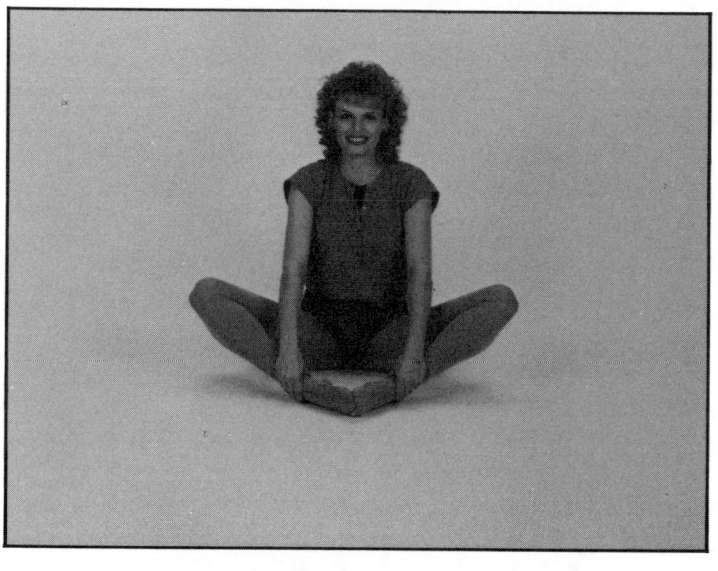

1 *Butterfly Variation:* Sit in a modified butterfly position with your toes together and heels apart.

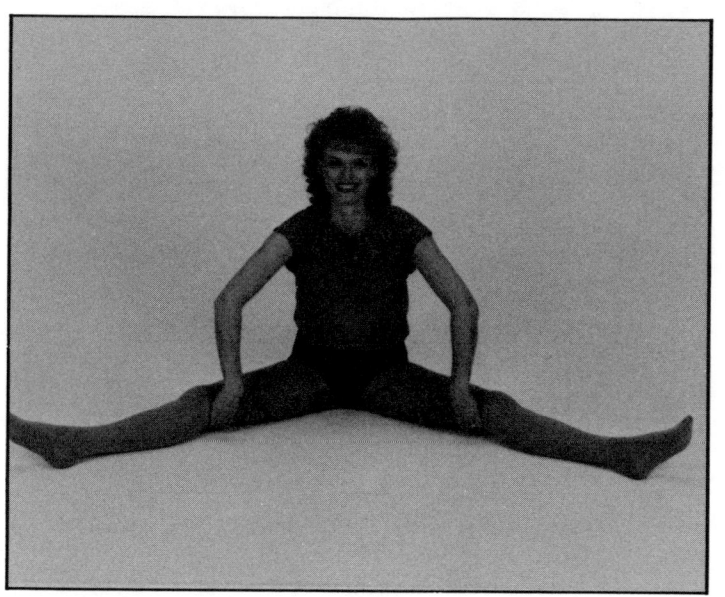

2 Open to straddle sit, and return to a modified butterfly position with toes together and heels apart. *Repetitions:* Repeat five times.

PRENATAL EXERCISES

Exercise No. 41

Lower Back Roll

Aim: To massage your lower back and stretch your inner thighs.

Starting Position: Back tuck.

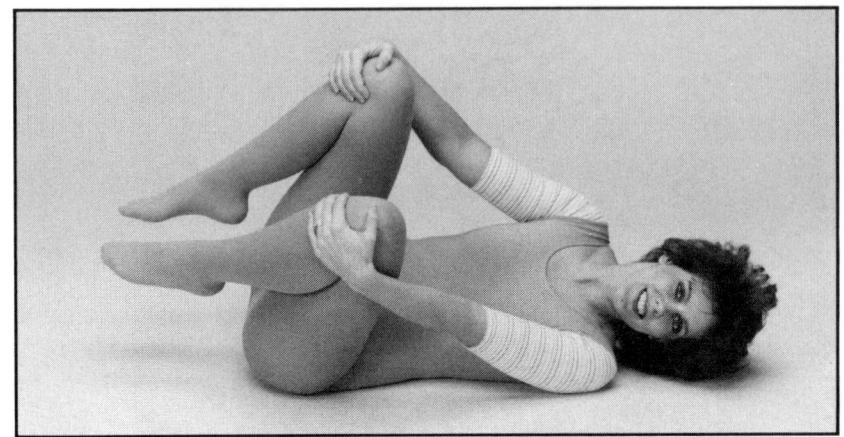

1 Slowly roll to the left.

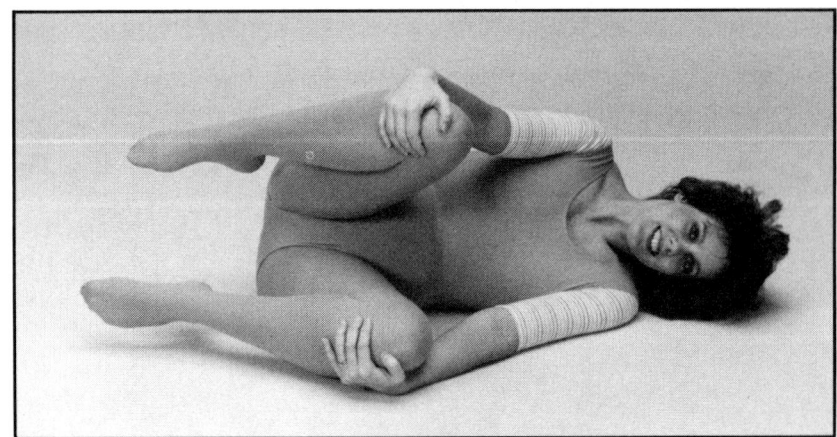

2 Open your legs far enough to feel a stretch in your inner thighs, and roll slowly to the right. *Repetitions:* Roll from side to side three to five times (the rolling motion will massage your lower back).

Note: If this exercise hurts your tailbone or bothers you in any way, do it more slowly or stop. You can try it again after your baby is born.

PRENATAL EXERCISES

Exercise No. 42

Knee Gliders

1. Bring your left knee over your right side, shifting your weight to your left hip as you do so.

2. Keeping your left knee on the floor, glide it toward your chest and back down until your leg is almost straight. *Repetitions:* Repeat three times on each side.

Aim: To relax your lower back, hips, and buttock muscles.

Starting Position: Lying on your right side with your head resting comfortably on your arm, and with your hips and knees slightly bent.

PRENATAL EXERCISES

Exercise No. 43

Body Relaxation

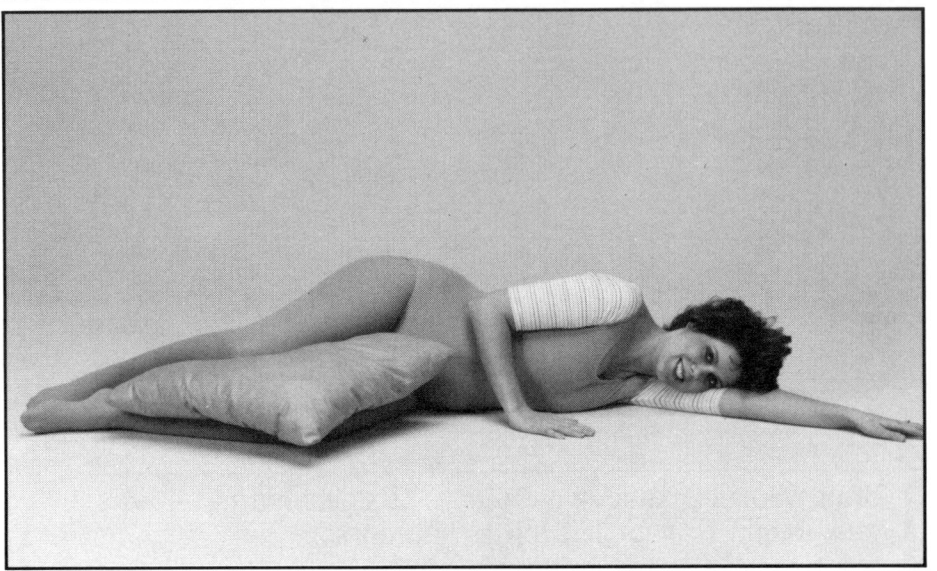

Aim: To relax you.

Starting Position: Lying on your left side.

1 Concentrate on something or somewhere very peaceful. Close your eyes and take deep breaths. In the following order, relax your *feet, legs, back, arms, neck, and face.* After you feel totally relaxed and peaceful, open your eyes, roll to all fours, and slowly stand up.

Note: Be sure to keep your face calm during this exercise. During delivery, many women distort their faces; doing this not only misplaces energy, but can result in broken capillaries in the face.

PRENATAL EXERCISES

Exercise No. 44

Elevate your feet above your heart, and rest for five to ten minutes. Roll to your side, sit for a moment to prevent light-headedness, then stand up. *Repetitions:* Try to elevate your legs for at least one-half hour per day, preferably for five or ten minutes in several sessions.

Leg Elevations

Aim: To prevent swelling and improve the circulation in your legs.

Starting Position: Hook-lying, resting on your elbows, or stacking pillows under your back for support.

Variation: While doing leg elevations, try exercise No. 45 (Finger Massage) to help pass the time.

Note: Your legs need to be elevated only above your heart.

PRENATAL EXERCISES

Exercise No. 45

Finger Massage

Aim: To improve circulation and help prevent swelling in your fingers and hands.

Starting Position: Any comfortable position.

1 Using your right hand to massage, start with the small finger of your left hand, and slowly bring each finger back as far as comfortably possible. Repeat, massaging your right hand with your left.

2 Using two fingers of your right hand, massage each finger on the left hand, pulling down from nail to knuckle. Repeat, massaging your left fingers with your right.

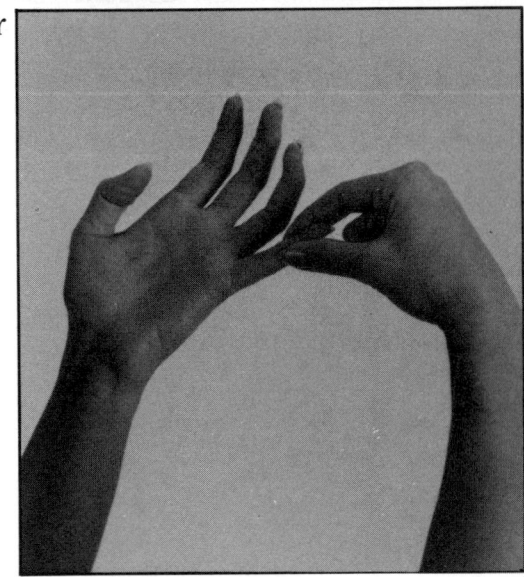

Chapter Two
Focus on Delivery

This chapter focuses on the period just before and just after the birth of your baby. It includes exercises to help you prepare for the possibility of a cesarean delivery and two sets of exercises to do in the hospital—one if you have given birth vaginally and the other if you have had a cesarean.

The best time to start your postpartum exercises is immediately after delivery or as soon as you feel up to it, provided your doctor has given his or her permission. You can begin getting back into shape while you are still in the hospital. Regardless of what kind of delivery you have, exercising within the first week after delivery helps relieve discomfort. To avoid any strain on your spine or any additional stretching of muscles, do the exercises in this chapter in your bed and use pillows to make yourself as comfortable as possible.

Human Relations

Labor is hard work. You can begin to prepare for getting the help you need during labor and delivery by encouraging your husband to read books about pregnancy and to participate with you in whatever prenatal classes or groups you are involved in. You need not be committed to any specific approach to delivery to benefit from the information and support that prenatal classes provide.

You and your husband also will probably want to learn about the possible complications of delivery that may require medical intervention (such as cesarean delivery) and special medications. Knowing about and discussing these issues together before delivery can help reduce the fear and mystery associated with them.

Another topic to focus on is breathing techniques. These techniques are not only crucial during delivery, but are also an important component of many prenatal exercises. A number of breathing exercises and techniques are covered in prenatal classes, as well as in many books about pregnancy and labor (see pages 15 to 17 in this book for breathing exercises).

After the delivery, you may be tempted to pay all of your attention to your newborn. As important as the new baby is, you and your partner deserve attention from one another as well.

Cesarean Delivery

Any unforeseen procedure such as an emergency cesarean can totally alter the experience of giving birth, but it need not destroy the beauty of the moment. When complications arise, the ability of a doctor to immediately reach your baby, if it becomes necessary, is a miraculous option for a healthy delivery.

A large percentage of cesarean deliveries are performed as emergencies. Many women find themselves unprepared because they haven't anticipated the possibility that a cesarean might be necessary to ensure a safe delivery in their particular situation. It is far better to be aware of the possibility of a surgical delivery than to be alarmed by the sudden necessity for one. Contact your hospital or doctor for information about cesarean delivery and classes in which cesarean birth is discussed.

Whether you know you will have a cesarean delivery or not, it is best to prepare for the possibility. The cesarean preparation exercise routine that follows is intended to help you to do so.

CESAREAN PREPARATION EXERCISES

Exercise No. 1

Simple Breaths

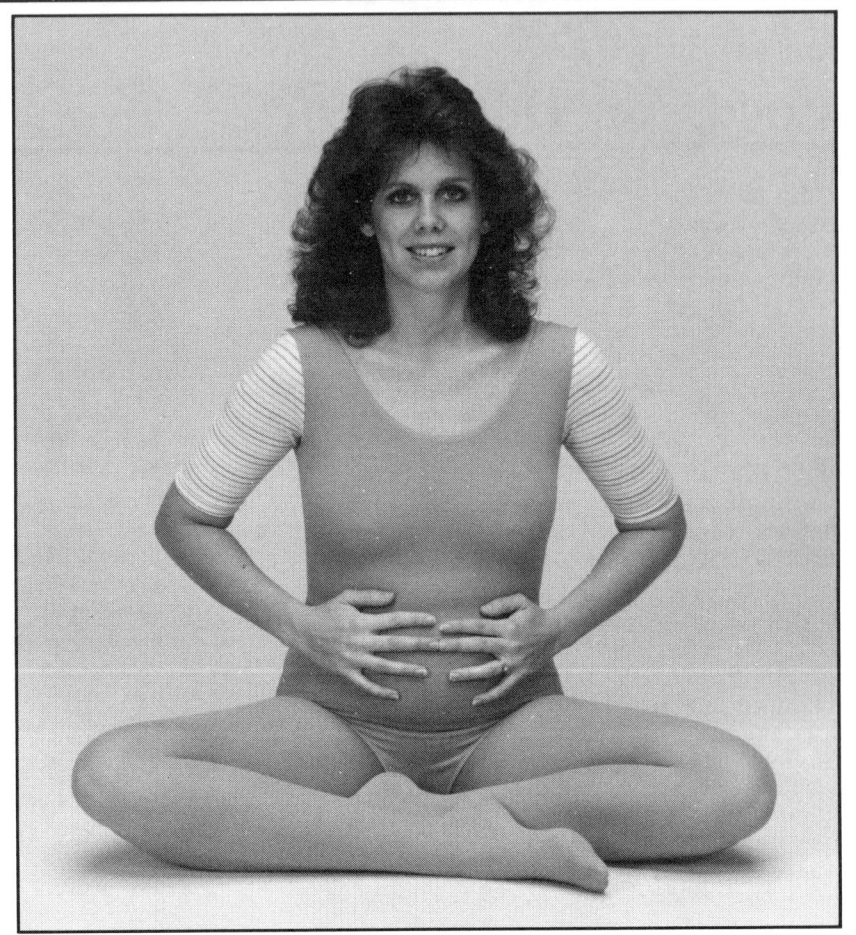

Aim: To teach you to breathe down into your diaphragm.

Starting Position: Tailor sit, with your hands on your stomach and the fingertips of your middle fingers touching lightly.

1 Breathing in through your nose, bring air into your lungs and allow it to push your stomach outward. Your fingertips should move apart slightly as your stomach expands. Hold your breath for a count of five, then slowly exhale (this will bring your fingertips back together). *Repetitions:* Repeat slowly three to five times.

CESAREAN PREPARATION EXERCISES

Exercise No. 2

Huffing/ Coughing

1 Press the sides of your hands firmly into your lower abdomen to practice supporting a vertical incision.

2 Press the sides of your hands firmly into your lower abdomen to practice supporting a horizontal incision.

3 *Huffing:* Change to a tailor sit. Breathe in deeply and sharply, then force air out and say "haa."
Coughing: Cough hard (if this is too difficult, continue to practice huffing).

Aim: To strengthen your diaphragm and make it easier to cough after surgery (particularly after receiving a general anesthetic).

Starting Position: Hook-lying.

CESAREAN PREPARATION EXERCISES

Exercise No. 3

Tuck and Pull

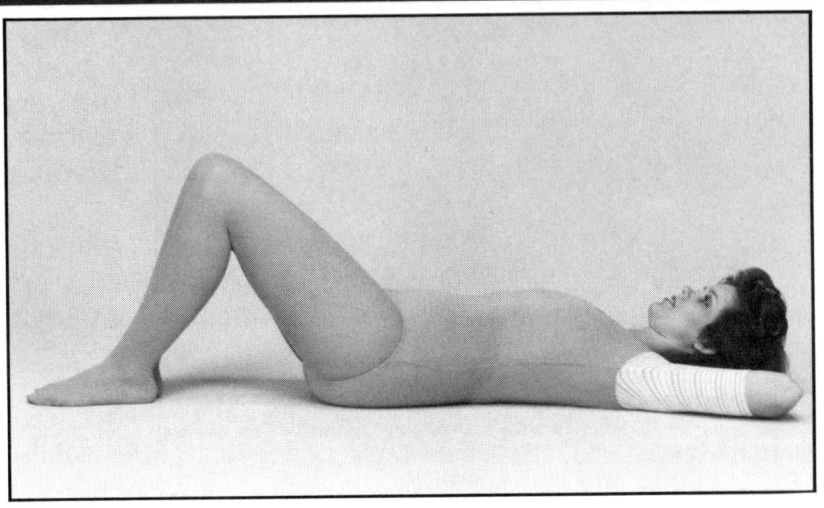

Aim: To strengthen your abdominal muscles and lengthen your lumbar muscles; also helps reduce backache.

Starting Position: Hook-lying or standing.

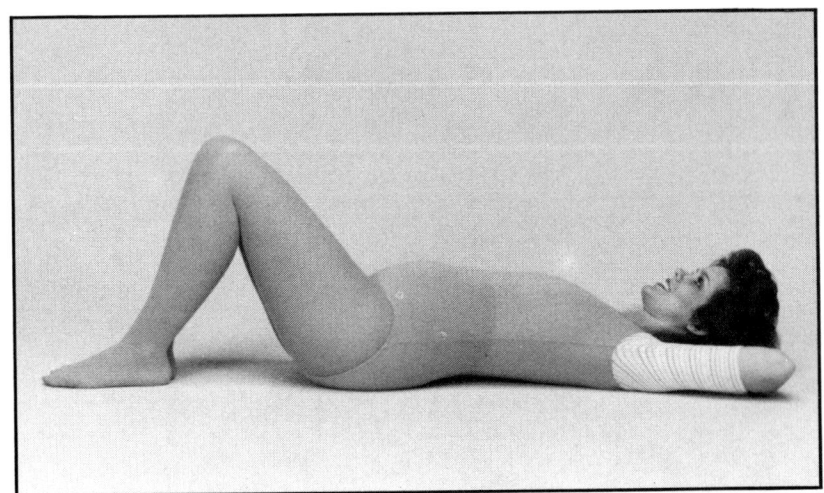

CESAREAN PREPARATION EXERCISES

Exercise No. 4

Leg and Foot Toner

Aim: To tone your leg and foot muscles and to improve your circulation; done daily, it can help prevent leg and foot cramps.

Starting Position: Pike sit with your palms flat on the floor behind you.

Point: Tighten your leg and buttock muscles, then point your toes, stretch, and pause. Relax. *Repetitions:* Repeat five times, then shake out your legs.

Flex: Point your toes toward the ceiling. Hold the position as you tighten your leg and buttock muscles, then relax. *Repetitions:* Repeat five times, then shake out your legs.

Circle: Keeping your feet flat on the floor, bend your knees, then lean back and rest on your forearms. Rest your left leg on your right knee and circle your left foot five times to the left, then five times to the right, flexing your foot and pointing your toes as you do so. *Repetitions:* Repeat with your right foot.

CESAREAN PREPARATION EXERCISES

Exercise Nos. 5 and 6

Kegels

Aim: To strengthen your pelvic floor muscles.

Starting Position: Standing, sitting, or lying down.

Note: Intermix kegels with other exercises during your exercise routine.

1 Tighten your vaginal and pelvic floor muscles as much as you can. Hold for a count of five, then relax. *Repetitions:* Repeat several times a day.

Leg Extenders (variation)

Aim: To strengthen your lower back, abdominal muscles, pectoral muscles, hamstrings, and buttock muscles.

Starting Position: Lying on your left side with your left knee slightly bent, your right leg extended, and resting your head on your left arm.

1 Bring your right knee toward your chest.

2 Slowly extend your right leg back to starting position. *Repetitions:* Repeat three to five times with right leg, then roll over to the right side and repeat three to five times with left leg.

CESAREAN PREPARATION EXERCISES

Exercise No. 7

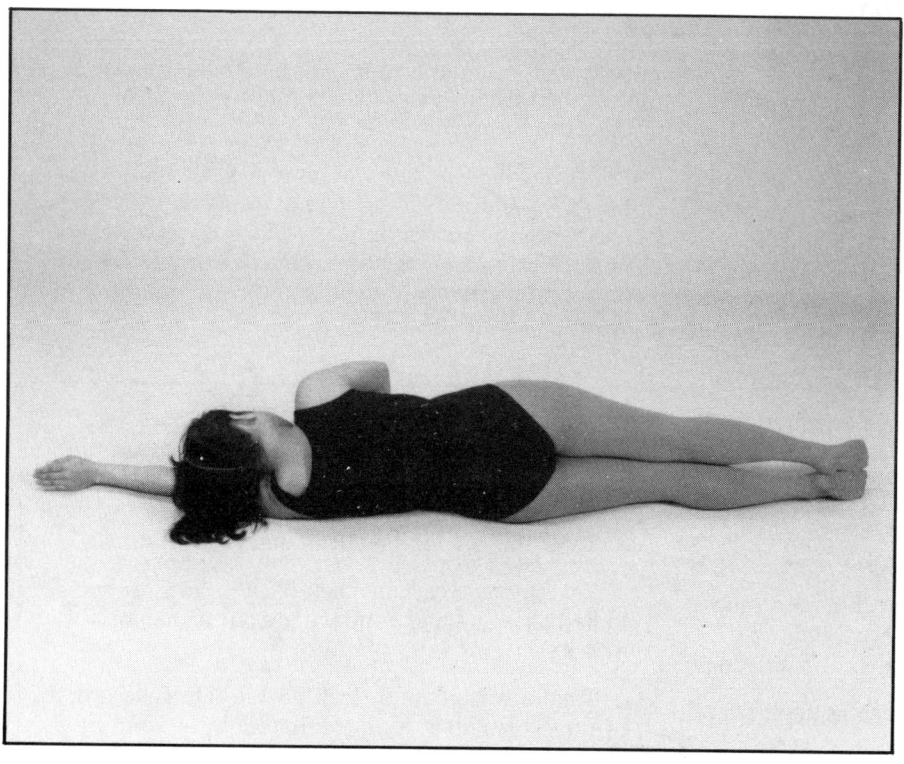

Tighten your buttock muscles. Hold this position for fifteen seconds, and then release. *Repetitions:* Repeat three to five times.

Cheek-to-Cheek

Aim: To tone your buttock muscles.

Starting Position: Lying on your left side with right leg directly on top of your left leg and knees slightly bent. Rest your head on your left arm and use your right arm in front to steady your body.

CESAREAN DELIVERY

Hospital Exercise Routine Following a Cesarean Delivery

Tightening your abdominal muscles slowly as soon after surgery as possible will help speed up your recovery.

After the delivery, take a couple of deep breaths, bend your feet, wiggle your toes, and tighten and relax your leg muscles. On your second or third day in the hospital, lie on your side with both your knees bent. This will encourage the natural progress of gas through your intestines. To help eliminate gas, lie on your side and massage your abdominal region to expel gas naturally. You can also try the breathing exercise described below under "Hints for Recovery from a Cesarean Delivery."

A day or two after you have started doing the deep breathing and muscle tightening exercises, add the postpartum exercises on pages 79 to 82. After you go home, continue doing these exercises on the floor or in bed to prepare you to start the postpartum exercise routine (pages 93 to 134).

Hints for Recovering from a Cesarean Delivery

- Do no heavy lifting for a minimum of three weeks following delivery. Limit lifting to ten to fifteen percent of your body weight.

- Before coughing, sneezing, or laughing, support the incision with your hands (see page 73).

- Nursing will speed your recovery, but your milk may be delayed for a couple of days. Find a comfortable position and have patience; it will come.

- Return to a regular fitness routine as soon after delivery as your doctor will allow.

- To help eliminate gas, lie on your side and massage your abdominal region to expel gas naturally. Try this exercise for gas pains:

1. Take a big breath in, then blow it out.

2. Take another big breath in and blow it out.

3. Take a big breath in, then blow it out slowly while tightening and contracting your abdominal muscles.

4. Take a big breath in and blow it out. Take two or three breaths at a time periodically, as soon as the first twinge of a gas pain appears.

CESAREAN DELIVERY: HOSPITAL EXERCISES

Exercise No. 1

Postpartum Breathing

Aim: To help you breathe down into your diaphragm.

Starting Position: Hook-lying in bed, with your legs slightly apart and your hands on your stomach with your fingertips touching.

Breathe in through your nose, bringing air into your diaphragm. Hold your breath to a count of five, then slowly exhale to a count of five. *Repetitions:* Repeat three or four times.

CESAREAN DELIVERY: HOSPITAL EXERCISES

Exercise No. 2

Leg and Foot Toner

Aim: To stretch and tone your legs and foot muscles and to improve your circulation; done daily, it can help prevent leg and foot cramps.

Starting Position: Lying flat on your back in bed, with a pillow under your knees.

1 *Point:* Point your toes and tighten your abdominal, leg, and buttock muscles. Relax. *Repetitions:* Repeat ten times. Shake out your legs.

2 *Flex:* Point your toes toward the ceiling. Flex one foot at a time. Hold the position, then relax. *Repetitions:* Repeat ten times. Shake out your legs.

3 *Circle:* In the same position, circle your right foot five times to the right, then five times to the left. *Repetitions:* Repeat with your left foot.

CESAREAN DELIVERY: HOSPITAL EXERCISES

Exercise Nos. 3 and 4

Bend your right knee slowly, then straighten it. Bend and straighten your left knee. *Repetitions:* Repeat five to ten times on each leg, alternating legs.

Knee Bends

Aim: To tone your legs.

Starting Position: Lying flat on your back in bed.

Tighten your vaginal and pelvic floor muscles as much as you can. Hold for a count of five, then relax. *Repetitions:* Repeat several times a day.

Kegels

Aim: To strengthen your pelvic floor muscles.

Starting Position: Lying in bed (or in the bathtub) in a comfortable position.

CESAREAN DELIVERY: HOSPITAL EXERCISES

Exercise Nos. 5 and 6

Pelvic Rock

Aim: To soothe your lower back and strengthen your abdominal muscles.

Starting Position: Hook-lying in bed, with your legs slightly apart and your arms at your sides.

Relax your back and press your lower back into the bed as you "tuck" your pelvis and contract your abdominal muscles. Relax. *Repetitions:* Repeat five times slowly.

Seat Squeeze

Aim: To strengthen your abdominal and buttock muscles and increase the flexibility of your back.

Starting Position: Hook-lying in bed, with your legs slightly apart and your arms at your sides.

"Tuck" your pelvis and contract your abdominal muscles while raising your hips off the bed, resting your weight on your shoulders. Tighten your buttock muscles as much as you can. Hold the position, then relax and slowly lower your hips to starting position. *Repetitions:* Repeat once.

VAGINAL DELIVERY

Hospital Exercise Routine Following a Vaginal Delivery

Most women experience labor-like contractions, called afterbirth pains, twenty-four to forty-eight hours after the birth of second or subsequent babies. If you are breastfeeding, the pains may be stronger. They can occur at any time, but especially each time you breastfeed your baby. Try the following breathing exercise when you are lying in bed to help relieve afterbirth pains and gas pains:

1. Take a big breath and blow it out.

2. Take another big breath and blow it out.

3. Take a third breath in and as you blow it out, contract your abdominal muscles.

4. Take a big breath and blow it out. Repeat the exercise two or three times, whenever you feel afterbirth pains or gas pains.

As soon as possible after delivery, start the hospital exercise routine on pages 84 to 89.

On the third day, continue with the exercises on pages 84 to 87 and add the following three exercises. After you're home, continue doing these exercises on the floor to prepare you to start the postpartum exercise routine.

VAGINAL DELIVERY

Exercise Nos. 1 and 2

Lying On Your Stomach

Aim: To help your uterus return to normal.

Starting Position: Lying on your stomach.

Note: For comfort, you may want to put a pillow under your chest and head, and rest on your folded arms.

Try to spend at least a half-hour per day on your stomach reading, sleeping, or relaxing.

Kegels

Aim: To strengthen your pelvic floor muscles.

Starting Position: Lying in bed (or in the bathtub) in a comfortable position.

Note: If you kegel each time you sit down, it will help you immensely in the weeks after delivery.

Note: The next day, continue to do these exercises, and add the following four exercises.

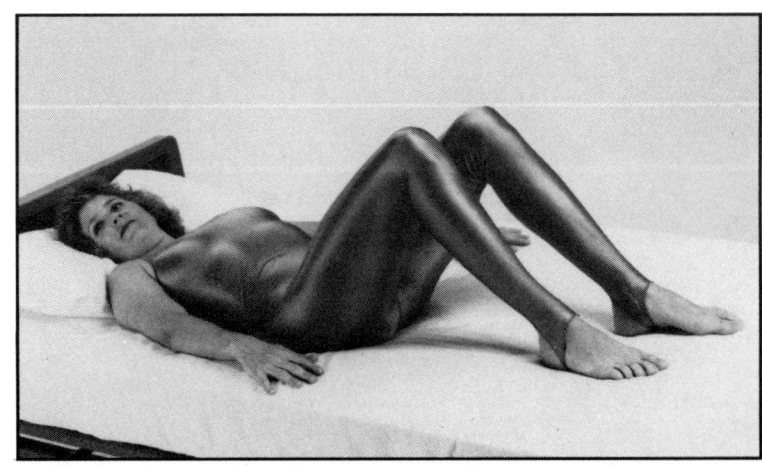

Tighten your vaginal and pelvic floor muscles as much as you can. Hold for a count of five, then relax. *Repetitions:* Repeat several times a day.

VAGINAL DELIVERY: HOSPITAL EXERCISES

Exercise Nos. 3 and 4

Postpartum Breathing

Breathe in through your nose, bringing air into your diaphragm. Hold your breath to a count of five, then slowly exhale to a count of five. *Repetitions:* Repeat three to five times.

Aim: To help you breathe down into your diaphragm.

Starting Position: Hook-lying in bed, with your legs slightly apart and your hands on your stomach with your fingertips touching.

Pelvic Rock

Relax your back and press your lower back into the bed as you "tuck" your pelvis and contract your abdominal muscles. Relax. *Repetitions:* Repeat five times slowly.

Aim: To soothe your lower back and strengthen your abdominal muscles.

Starting Position: Hook-lying in bed, with your legs slightly apart and your arms at your sides.

VAGINAL DELIVERY: HOSPITAL EXERCISES

Exercise No. 5

Knee Bends

Aim: To tone your legs.

Starting Position: Lying flat on your back in bed.

Bend your right knee slowly, then straighten it. Bend and straighten your left knee. *Repetitions:* Repeat five to ten times on each leg, alternating legs.

VAGINAL DELIVERY: HOSPITAL EXERCISES

Exercise No. 6

Leg and Foot Toner

1 *Point:* Point your toes and tighten your abdominal, leg, and buttock muscles. Relax. *Repetitions:* Repeat ten times. Shake out your legs.

2 *Flex:* Point your toes toward the ceiling. Flex one foot at a time. Hold the position, then relax. *Repetitions:* Repeat ten times. Shake out your legs.

Aim: To stretch and tone your leg and foot muscles and to improve your circulation; done daily, it can help prevent leg and foot cramps.

Starting Position: Lying flat on your back in bed, with a pillow under your knees.

3 *Circle:* In the same position, circle your right foot five times to the right, then five times to the left. *Repetitions:* Repeat with your left foot.

VAGINAL DELIVERY: HOSPITAL EXERCISES

Exercise Nos. 7 and 8

Back Tucks

Aim: To strengthen your lower back and buttock muscles.

Starting Position: Lying flat on your back in bed.

Keeping your back flat on the bed, bring one knee up close to your chest and grasp it with your arms, then slowly lower your leg. *Repetitions:* Repeat five times with each leg, alternating legs.

Seat Squeeze

Aim: To strengthen your abdominal and buttock muscles and increase the flexibility of your back.

Starting Position: Hook-lying in bed, with your legs slightly apart and your arms at your sides.

"Tuck" your pelvis and pull your abdominal muscles in while raising your hips off the bed, resting your weight on your shoulders. Tighten your buttock muscles as much as you can. Hold the position, then relax and slowly lower your hips to starting position. *Repetitions:* Repeat once.

VAGINAL DELIVERY: HOSPITAL EXERCISES

Exercise No. 9

1 Draw your right leg to your chest.

2 Extend your right leg toward the ceiling, pointing your toes. Press your lower back to the bed.

3 Flex your right foot and lower your leg slowly to the bed. *Repetitions:* Repeat three times with each leg, alternating legs.

Leg Raisers

Aim: To strengthen your abdominal and buttock muscles, lower back, and legs.

Starting Position: Hook-lying.

Note: After you are home, continue this exercise routine on the floor to prepare you to start the postpartum exercise routine (pages 91 to 134).

Chapter Three
Postpartum Concerns and Exercise Routine

This chapter begins with a discussion of what postpartum adjustment means to both you and your husband and concludes with a postpartum exercise routine that you can begin when you come home from the hospital.

Human Relations

The difficulties of adjusting to a new baby can make the weeks following delivery a very stressful time for the whole family. During the postpartum period, the stress of learning to cope with the demands of a newborn, magnified by being in a state of chronic fatigue, can cause your self-esteem to hit bottom. At the same time, your husband may feel left out, neglected, and jealous of the baby. These feelings, perhaps compounded by fears that he will harm the seemingly delicate baby, can lower his self-esteem as well. When both parents feel this way, the result can be a combination of anger and despair.

This is not to stress the negative aspects of postpartum family life, but rather to emphasize the importance of sharing your concerns with each other during this sometimes trying period. It may help to remember that what all the members of the family need most at this time is caring attention from one another.

Some experts say that the postpartum mother herself needs mothering. Your ability to become attached to and care for your baby may be determined in part by the love and caring you receive from others. Therefore, your husband must be sensitive to this need and make the extra effort to be with you and to support you with his words and deeds.

One study of "postpartum blues" recommends that the new mother take time to relax and separate herself from the events of the day, every day. In order to do this, you will have to ask for help from others, and especially from your husband. It is important that you learn to do so, for by caring for yourself—whether by napping while your husband cares for the baby, soaking in a hot bath, or going shopping for an hour—you will be caring for those close to you, including your baby.

Your husband needs special attention as well. To counteract feelings of being left out, he can take care of the baby for short periods of time when you are not present. By helping out in this way, he can reduce the burden on you while he builds up his competence as a parent. Contact with the baby will also reduce any fears he may have about the delicacy of the newborn, and will help him feel close to both the baby and you. If your husband is feeling neglected from a lack of sexual contact, he may need to discover closeness that is possible without intercourse.

It is also important that you make time to be together as a couple, without your baby. Arranging for competent baby-sitting help will help improve your physical and mental health. Another study of postpartum blues found that among the keys to successful readjustment were continuing to socialize as a couple, though less often than before, and continuing outside interests while limiting outside responsibilities.

The key to getting through the postpartum adjustment period is to share your feelings with your partner

POSTPARTUM CONCERNS

and to decide together how to work out problems, instead of holding anger and resentment inside.

A first step might be for you and your husband to talk about what each of you knows and doesn't know about the baby. There is no assurance in our society today that either parent knows anything about caring for a newborn. Your role as parents is just beginning; every few months for the next twenty years, your child will probably present you with a new mystery to solve. The challenge to you and your husband is to learn together and to ask for help.

There is more help available to parents than they usually recognize. Abundant advice can be had not only from books, but also from pediatricians and counselors, teachers and youth workers, and other parents. Sometimes parents lack the self-confidence to ask questions and to seek help; or they may believe that if they join a parenting group, they will be admitting to some fault on their part. Parents need to recognize that it is natural to seek training in the important task of child-rearing. The result will be healthier parents, children, and families.

Postpartum Exercise Routine

After nine months, you probably can't wait to get back into your "normal" clothes. Then, to your disappointment, you find that the dimensions of your hips have changed dramatically, leftover pounds remain to be lost, and your stomach still looks pregnant.

Many women trace lifelong weight problems back to not getting their bodies back into shape after pregnancy. Gynecologists say that doing exercises to strengthen the pelvic floor during and after pregnancy helps prevent possible prolapse of the uterus (i.e., sliding of the uterus down into the vaginal canal) later in life. It is extremely important to get back into shape as soon after your child's birth as possible by following a program of exercises to strengthen the pelvic floor area. Although your baby's first year of life is a very busy time for you, any delay in taking care of yourself will likely backfire. An out-of-shape, unhappy woman is not as effective a mother as she could be.

As you begin this exercise routine, remember that, first and foremost, you must have patience. You can get back into shape, lose weight, and firm up by exercising —but it won't happen instantly. Also, you may not return to your prepregnancy dimensions or weight, particularly if you are nursing. If you are nursing, add five to ten pounds to your target weight to compensate for retained fluids, etc. This is called your "nursing weight." The time to lose additional weight is after you have finished nursing your baby.

Your postpartum exercise routine will be easier if you have exercised during pregnancy. Be sure to check with your doctor before you start any exercise program. It is extremely important to be sure you have healed and that any bleeding has stopped before doing this postpartum exercise routine.

To chart your progress, you may want to record your weight and measurements when you start, check them six weeks later, and then check them periodically for the next year. Remember—start slowly, then gradually work up to your target heart rate and down to your target weight. And enjoy every little sign of progress!

Note: If you are using this book on your own, rather than in conjunction with a You & Me, Baby exercise class, you'll benefit most from the postpartum exercise routine if you perform it at least three times a week. The exercises are intended to be performed in the order in which they are presented here.

POSTPARTUM EXERCISES

Exercise No. 1

1. Start walking slowly, then lengthen your stride, swinging your arms in an exaggerated motion. Maintain a breathe-relax, breathe-relax rhythm.

Walking

Aim: To slowly "waken" your body by loosening up your muscles through a series of relaxed leg exercises combined with arm work.

Starting Position: Standing.

2. Alternately raise your right and left knees as you walk, to help loosen your hip flexor muscles.

Note: As you walk more briskly, add the arm exercises on the next page.

POSTPARTUM EXERCISES

Exercise No. 2

Walking– Arm Exercises

Aim: To slowly "waken" your body by loosening up your muscles through a series of relaxed leg exercises combined with arm work.

Starting Position: Walking with arms in cross position, palms up.

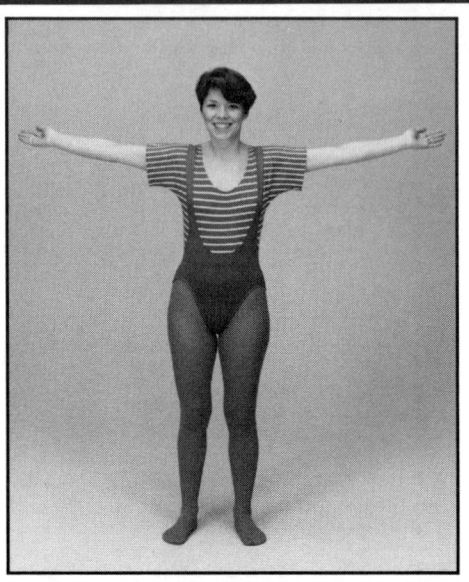

1 Extend your arms at shoulder level.

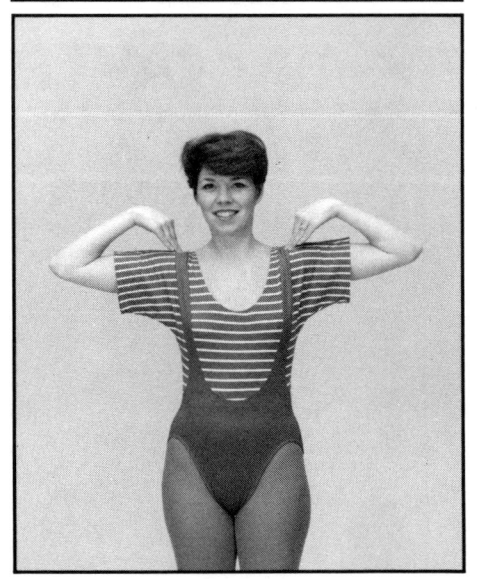

2 Bend your elbows and touch your shoulders.

POSTPARTUM EXERCISES

3 Cross your hands over your head to touch opposite ears.

1 *Variation:* From starting position, bend your elbows and touch your shoulders.

4 Return your hands to your shoulders and extend your arms again. *Repetitions:* Repeat quickly, to a count of four.

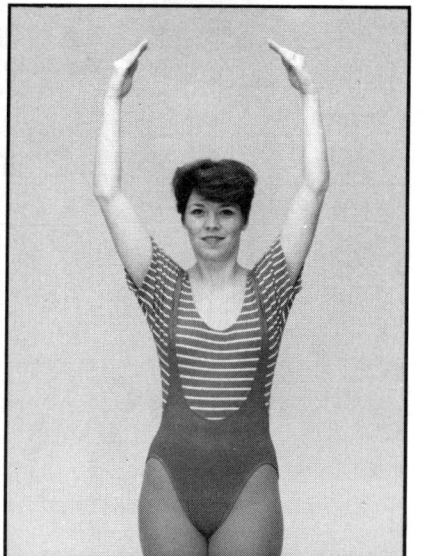

2 Extend your arms upward. Lower them, touch your shoulders, and return to starting position. *Repetitions:* Repeat quickly to a count of four.

POSTPARTUM EXERCISES

Exercise No. 3

Start-Up Stretch

Aim: To loosen up your arms and shoulders and stretch your lower back.

Starting Position: Standing, with your feet shoulder-width apart, your knees bent, and your toes and knees aligned.

1 Place your hands on your upper anterior thighs and press your right shoulder toward your left shoulder.

2 Repeat, pressing your left shoulder toward your right shoulder. *Repetitions:* Repeat ten times to each side, alternating.

POSTPARTUM EXERCISES

Exercise No. 4

Knee Lifts

Aim: To stretch the gluteal and hamstring muscles.

Starting Position: Standing comfortably, with your feet two to three feet apart and arms in a cross position.

1 Lift knees high in front, alternate right and left.

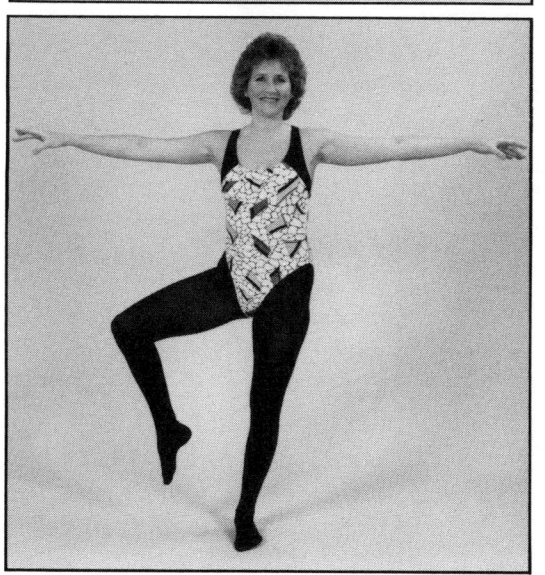

2 Keeping arms in cross position, lift knees high to the side, alternating right and left. *Repetitions:* Repeat the entire exercise for two sets of four knee lifts, alternating right and left.

POSTPARTUM EXERCISES

Exercise No. 5

Raggedy Ann

Aim: To loosen up and relax your body, particularly your neck, shoulders, and legs. This exercise can be done at any time during the exercise routine.

Starting Position: Standing erect with your feet shoulder-width apart, your knees bent, and your toes and knees aligned.

1 Press your left palm toward the ceiling, stretching the entire left side of your body until your left heel rises slightly off the floor. *Repetitions:* Repeat on your right side, then on your left side, then again on your right side.

2 With your knees slightly bent, round your shoulders and raise your arms to shoulder level. Alternately press forward with your left hand, then with your right hand, as if pushing an object away.

3 Keeping your hips in with your shoulders, drop your head forward with your chin to your chest. Round your shoulders forward, bend your knees, and roll up to starting position. *Repetitions:* Repeat the entire exercise one to three times.

POSTPARTUM EXERCISES

Exercise No. 6

1 *Shoulder Rotations:* Raise your shoulders to your ears. Pull your shoulders back and downward, then up and forward.

Shoulders

2 With your left shoulder, "draw" three circles forward, then three circles backward. Repeat with your right shoulder. Draw three circles forward with both shoulders, then reverse and draw three circles backward.

Aim: To loosen up your shoulders and tone your upper arms.

Starting Position: Standing with your feet slightly apart and your arms at your sides; may also be done sitting.

1 *Shoulder Lifts:* Lift your shoulders and roll them forward. With your palms facing out, bring your arms forward until your little fingers touch.

2 Lift your shoulders again and roll them backwards. With your palms still facing out, bring your arms behind your body until you feel the stretch in your shoulders. *Repetitions:* Repeat three times.

POSTPARTUM EXERCISES

Exercise No. 6

Shoulders

Aim: To loosen up your shoulders and tone your upper arms.

Starting Position: Standing with your feet slightly apart and your arms at your sides; may also be done sitting.

Note: Never drop your head and shoulders to the back.

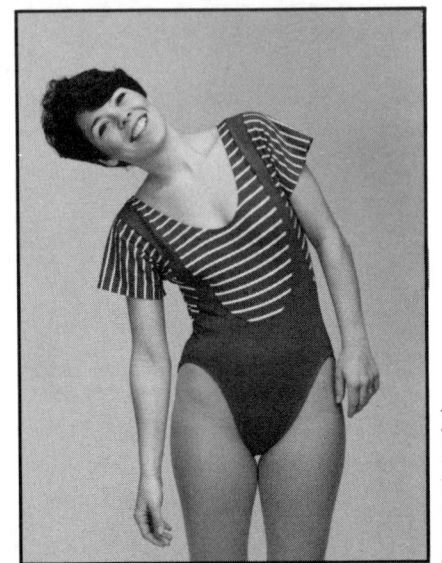

1 *Triangles:* Tuck your pelvis in and pull in your abdominal muscles. Keep them tucked throughout this exercise. Lean your head and right shoulder to the right.

2 Roll both shoulders forward and let your head drop forward slightly. Extend your arms down in front of you with the backs of your hands touching.

3 Lean your head and shoulders to the left. Return to starting position. *Repetitions:* Repeat three times, alternating from left to right.

POSTPARTUM EXERCISES
Exercise No. 7

Head Arcs

Aim: To loosen up your neck and shoulders.

Starting Position: Standing, with your feet slightly apart and your arms at your sides. This exercise may also be done sitting.

1 Drop your left ear to your left shoulder; return to starting position. Drop your right ear to your right shoulder; return to starting position.

2 Roll your chin to your chest and back up again.

3 Turn your head to look left, then right. *Repetitions:* Repeat three times.

POSTPARTUM EXERCISES

Exercise No. 8

Face Exercises

Aim: To tighten your face muscles.

Starting Position: Standing, with your feet slightly apart and your arms at your sides. This exercise may also be done sitting.

1 Smile.

2 Pucker your face; then relax.

Note: Also try exercising your face by chewing gum and forming vowel sounds or words with your mouth.

POSTPARTUM EXERCISES

Exercise No. 9

Arm Series

Arm Circles: With your palms up, move your arms forward to make five to ten small circles, then five to ten large circles. *Repetitions:* Repeat moving your arms backward, then repeat with your palms down.

Aim: To strengthen your upper and lower arms, wrists, and pectoral muscles.

Starting Position: Standing with your feet shoulders'-width apart and your arms in cross position.

Wrist Flexors: Moving only your wrists, point your fingertips toward the ceiling, then toward the floor. *Repetitions:* Repeat five to ten times.

Scarecrow: With palms down, spread your fingers. Bend your arms at the elbows and swing palms in front of your body. Return to starting position. *Repetitions:* Repeat five to ten times.

Back Sweeper: With palms down, spread your fingers. Bend your arms at the elbows and try to touch your fingertips behind your back. Return to starting position. *Repetitions:* Repeat five to ten times slowly.

POSTPARTUM EXERCISES

Exercise No. 9

Arm Series

Aim: To strengthen your upper and lower arms, wrists, and pectoral muscles.

Starting Position: Standing with your feet shoulder-width apart and arms in a cross position.

1 *Elbow Flex:* With your palms up, make fists.

2 Bend your elbows until your fists touch your shoulders, then circle forearms downward and outward until extended.

3 Turn your fists toward the ceiling.

4 Bend your elbows and touch your fists to your shoulders, then return to starting position. *Repetitions:* Repeat entire exercise five times.

POSTPARTUM EXERCISES

Exercise No. 9

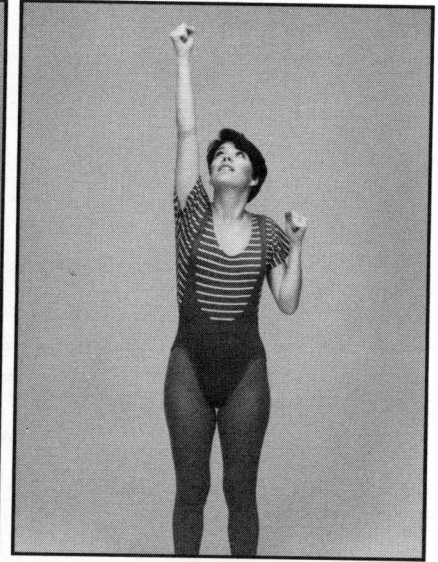

1 *Arm Punches:* Make fists. Punch forward five to ten times, alternating arms.

2 Punch over your head five to ten times, alternating arms.

3 Punch out to your sides five to ten times, alternating arms.

Push Backs: Turn your palms away from you and gently push up and back. *Repetitions:* Repeat five to ten times.

POSTPARTUM EXERCISES

Exercise No. 9

Arm Series

Aim: To strengthen your upper and lower arms, wrists, and pectoral muscles.

Starting Position: Standing, with your feet shoulder-width apart and your arms in cross position.

Scissors: Hold your arms straight in front of your body, with your palms down. Move your arms in a scissors motion, alternating right over left arm and left over right arm. *Repetitions:* Repeat the entire exercise with your palms up ten times and with your palms down ten times.

Elbows Together: Bend your arms at the elbows. Tightening your arms, make fists, and bring your forearms together in front of your body. Press your arms open to cross position.
Repetitions: Repeat five to ten times.

POSTPARTUM EXERCISES

Exercise No. 10

Skier's Sit

Aim: To strengthen your legs, abdominal muscles, and lower back.

Starting Position: Standing with your back against a wall.

1. Bend your knees and slide your upper body down. "Sit" with your thighs at a right angle to the wall, as if you were sitting on a stool. Press the small of your back firmly against the wall. (This is a great time to practice kegels.) Hold the position for twenty to forty-five seconds.

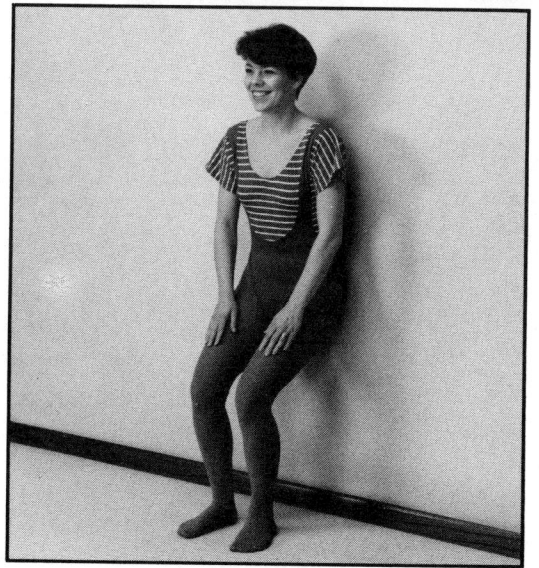

2. Lean forward and place your hands on your knees, then slowly straighten your back. Straighten your knees slowly and return to a standing position.

POSTPARTUM EXERCISES

Exercise No. 11

Leg Lifts

Aim: To tone your leg muscles.

Starting Position: Standing at a wall, with your left palm resting comfortably against the wall, or standing beside a chair, with your left hand resting on the back of the chair.

1 Draw your right knee up toward your chest, keeping your back straight. Circle your right foot five times in each direction.

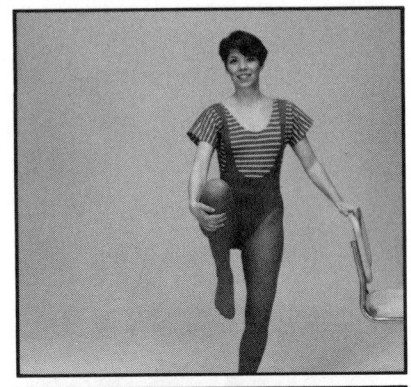

2 Keeping your left knee slightly bent, draw your right knee to your right side.

3 Drop your right leg to a comfortable position and straighten it. Bend and straighten your right leg ten times. *Repetitions:* Repeat the entire exercise with your left leg.

POSTPARTUM EXERCISES

Exercise No. 12

Calf Stretch

Aim: To stretch your calf muscles in preparation for walking.

Starting Position: Standing an arm's length from the wall, palms flat against the wall, toes pointed forward, and hips pressed forward.

1 Step forward with your right foot, bending your right knee, and stretching your left leg behind you (keep both heels on the floor). Keeping your lower back flat, hold a comfortable stretch for fifteen seconds. Do not bounce. Return to starting position. *Repetitions:* Repeat with your left foot forward.

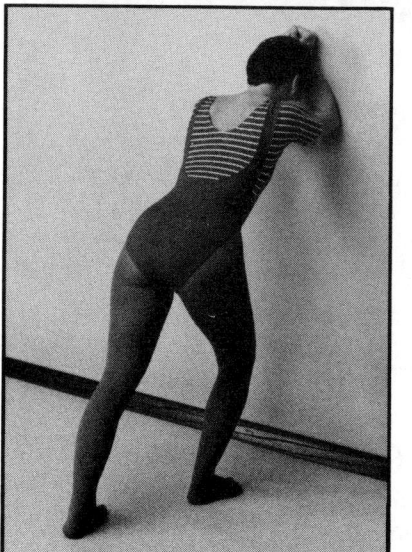

2 *Variation:* As you stretch, lean forward and rest your head on your hands.

POSTPARTUM EXERCISES

Exercise No. 13

Walking/ Jogging

Aim: To strengthen your cardiovascular system and your legs.

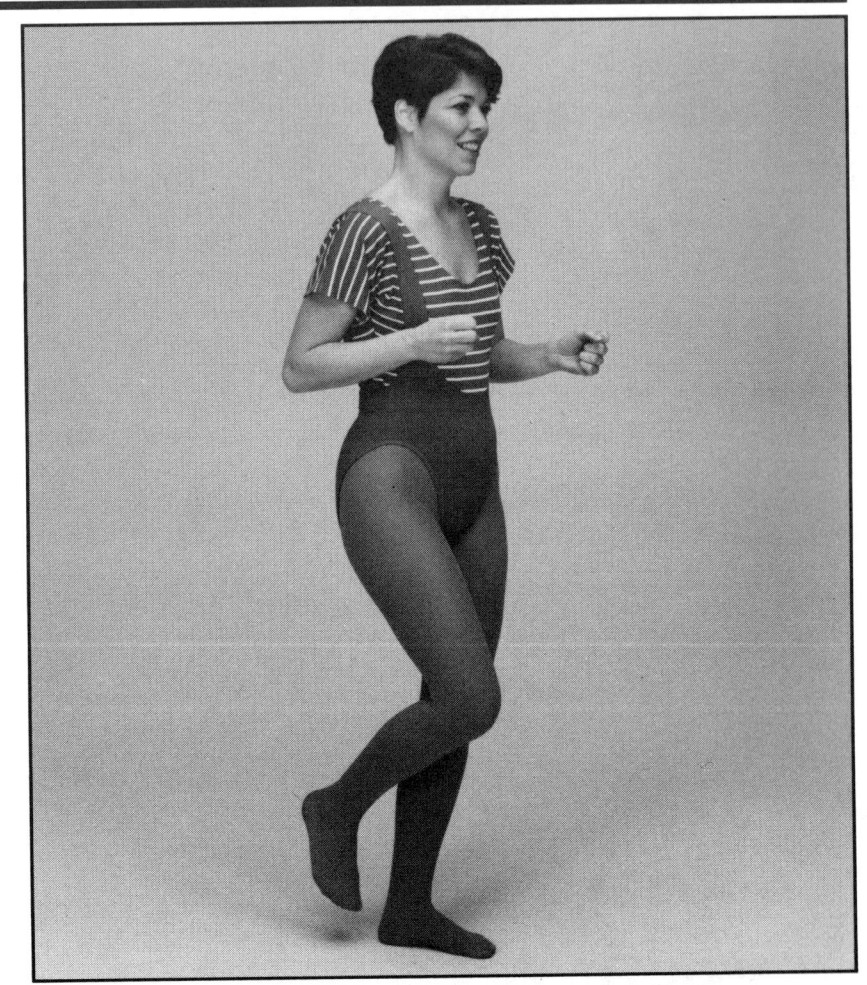

1 Walk briskly or jog. Strive for fifteen to twenty minutes with your heart rate between fifty and seventy percent of your maximum target heart rate. (See pages 8 to 10 for information about the cardiovascular system and target heart rate.)

POSTPARTUM EXERCISES

Exercise No. 14

Side Lean

Aim: To trim your waistline.

Starting Position: Standing two or three feet from a wall, holding left arm out at shoulder height with left palm flat against the wall.

1 Raise your right arm over your head and lock your left elbow. Stretch your right side by reaching over your head with your right arm, pushing your hips out slightly, away from the wall. Try to touch your right hand to the wall.

2 Lower your right arm and lean your hips toward the wall (be sure to keep your left arm locked). *Repetitions:* Repeat entire exercise three to five times on each side.

POSTPARTUM EXERCISES

Exercise No. 15

Plié Series

Aim: To tone your legs, waist, buttock muscles, and lower back.

Starting Position: Standing erect with your feet shoulder-width apart, with your pelvis tucked, your abdominal muscles pulled in, your knees bent, and your toes and knees aligned.

1 *Side-to-Side Sway:* Sway from side to side, keeping your hips and shoulders in vertical alignment. *Repetitions:* Repeat five times, alternating sides.

2 *Stride Sway:* Keeping your feet shoulder-width apart, take one step forward with your left foot. Sway forward and back, keeping your heels on the floor. *Repetitions:* Repeat ten times with each foot, then return to starting position and repeat the *side-to-side sway* five times.

3 *Elbow-hip sway:* Place your hands on your shoulders and lower your right elbow to your right hip, then return to upright position. Lower your left elbow to your left hip, then return to upright position. *Repetitions:* Repeat ten times, alternating sides. Return to starting position and repeat the *side-to-side sway* five times.

POSTPARTUM EXERCISES

Exercise No. 16

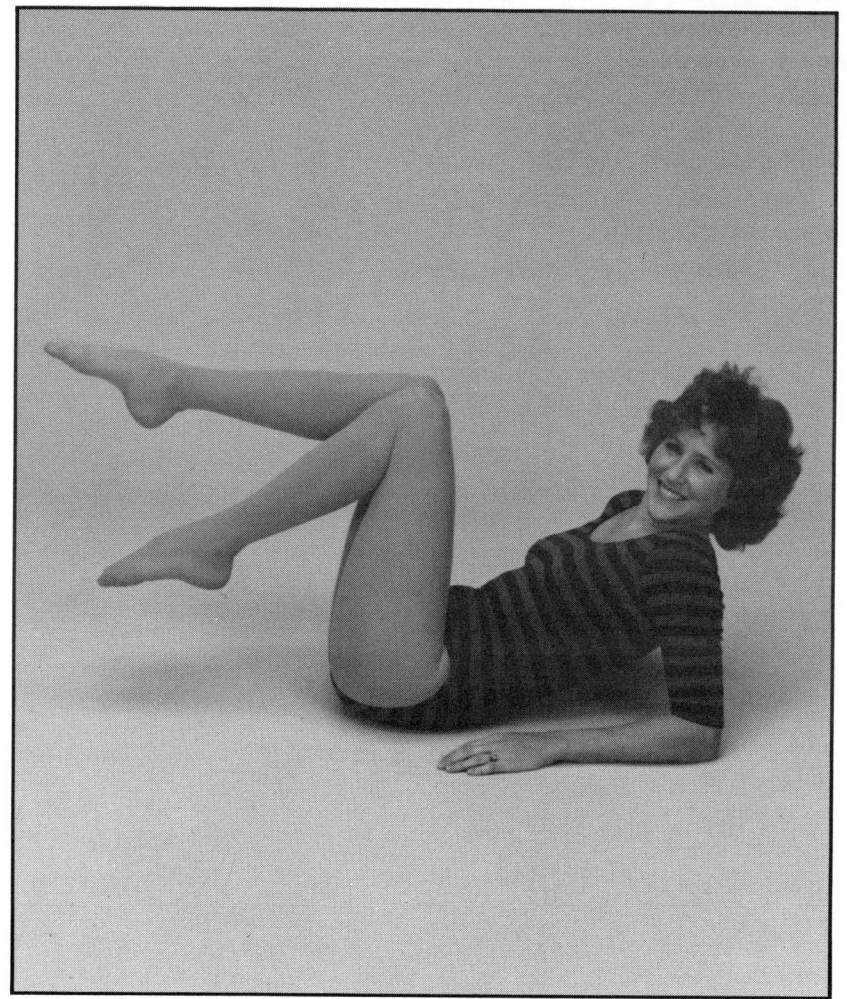

Bicycles on Elbows

Aim: To strengthen your abdomen and lower back muscles, and to increase the circulation in and mobility of your legs.

Starting Position: Hook-lying, supporting your upper-body weight on your elbows.

Bicycle forward and reverse for thirty seconds. Rest, then bicycle another thirty seconds. *Repetitions:* Work up to a full five to ten minutes of bicycling (a kitchen timer may be helpful).

Note: This is a fun exercise to do side-by-side with your baby because the baby will try to imitate your movements.

POSTPARTUM EXERCISES

Exercise No. 17

Seat Squeeze

Aim: To strengthen your abdominal and buttock muscles and increase the flexibility of your back.

Starting Position: Hook-lying, with your feet slightly apart.

1 "Tuck" your pelvis and pull your abdominal muscles in while raising your hips slightly off the floor, resting your weight on your shoulders. Tighten your buttocks as much as you can, then release. Slowly lower your hips to the floor to starting position. *Repetitions:* Repeat five times.

2 With your feet still apart, put your knees together, "tuck" your pelvis, and pull in your abdominal muscles. Raise your hips, then tighten and release your buttock muscles. Lower your hips to the floor to starting position. *Repetitions:* Repeat five times.

3 Put your knees and feet together and raise your hips, then tighten and release your buttock muscles. Lower your hips to the floor to starting position. *Repetitions:* Repeat five times.

Note: To avoid putting pressure on your neck, do not raise your hips too high.

POSTPARTUM EXERCISES

Exercise No. 18

Abdominal Series

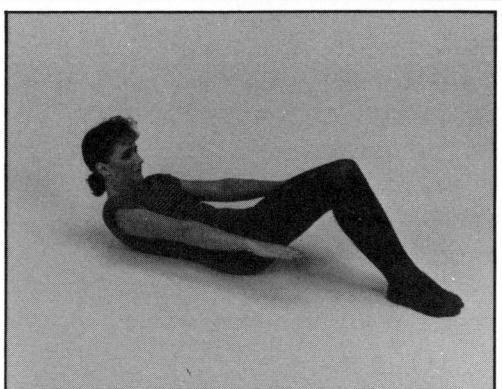

Curl-Ups: Starting position #1 or #2. Lie on your back, with your knees bent, keeping your feet flat on the floor. Curl up slowly (don't jerk), just far enough for your shoulder blades to come off the floor. Hold your head and neck tight, in a fixed position. Lower to starting position. *Note:* Hold your chin to your chest when curling up.
Repetitions: Start with five and work up to thirty or more.

1 *Diastasis Variation:* Starting position #3. Slowly curl down to the floor, with your chin on your chest, placing one vertebra on the floor at a time.

2 Roll to your right side; then return to starting position. Repeat step 1; then roll to your left side.
Repetitions: Repeat the entire exercise ten times.

Aim: To strengthen your abdominal muscles and lower back.

Starting Positions: #1. Hook-lying, with your arms crossed, holding your ribs. #2. Hook-lying, with your arms bent and your fingers locked or hands crossed on top of your head. #3. Sitting with your knees to your chest and hugging your ribs, crossing your arms over your abdomen for support.

POSTPARTUM EXERCISES

Exercise No. 18

Abdominal Series

Aim: To strengthen your oblique abdominal muscles.

Starting Position: If you have a separated rectus diastasis muscle, use starting position #1 on page 115. Otherwise, use starting position #2 on page 115.

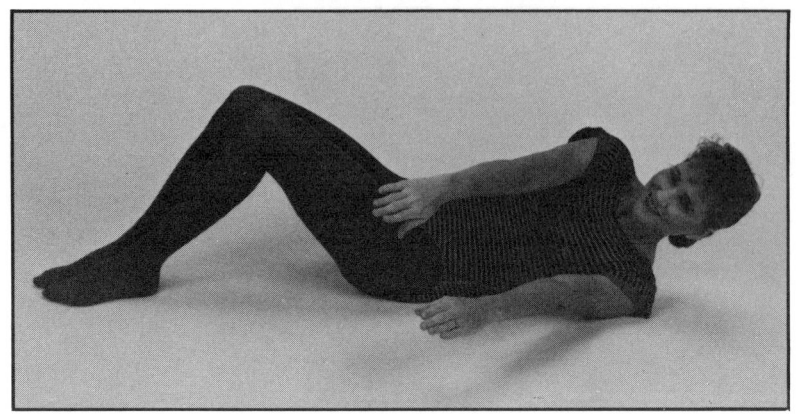

1 *Oblique Variation:* Curl up, lifting your right shoulder. Point your right elbow toward your left knee, and curl back down. Repeat.

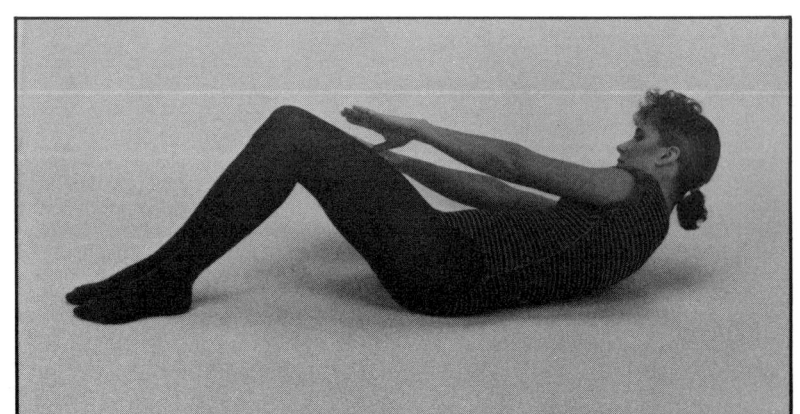

2 Curl up, lifting your left shoulder. Point your left elbow toward your right knee, and curl back down.
Repetitions: Start with five on each side, alternating, and work up to twenty (ten on each side) or more.

POSTPARTUM EXERCISES

Exercise No. 19

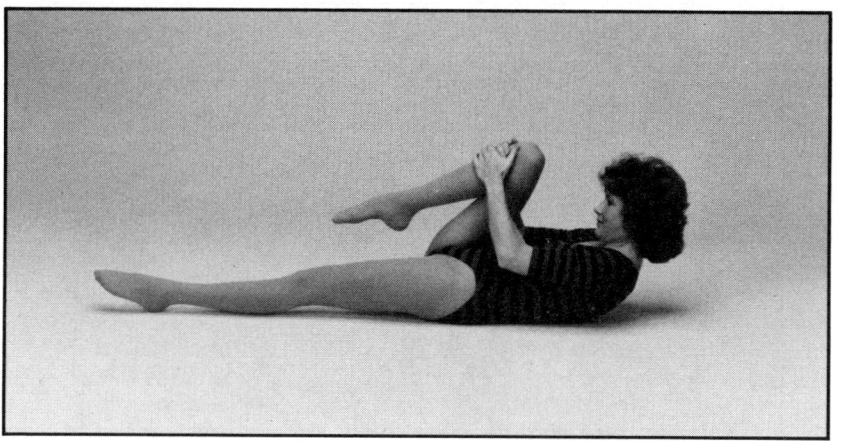

1 Raise your head and shoulders off the floor. Bring your right knee to your chest and grasp it. As you release your right leg, bring your left knee to your chest and grasp it. *Repetitions:* Repeat five times with each leg, alternating legs.

Back Tucks

Aim: To strengthen your abdominal muscles and stretch your lower back muscles.

Starting Position: Lying flat on your back with your arms at your sides.

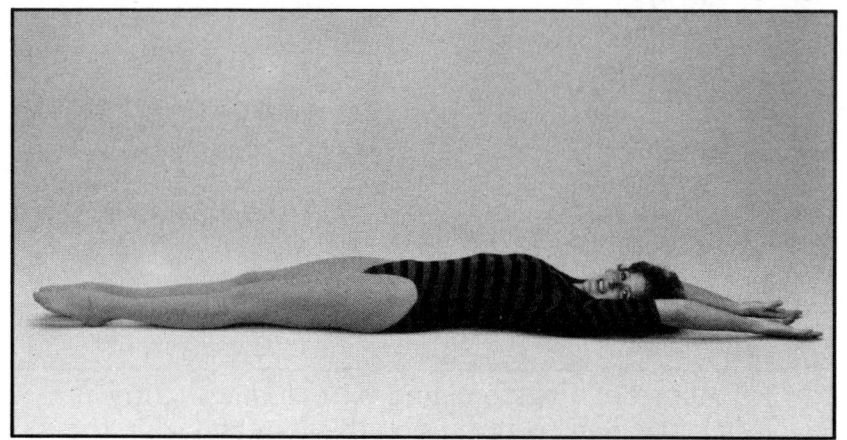

2 Return to starting position. Raise your arms above your head, point your toes, and stretch. *Repetitions:* Repeat the entire exercise two to four times.

POSTPARTUM EXERCISES

Exercise No. 20

Sitting Tucks

Aim: To tighten your abdominal muscles and tone your entire body.

Starting Position: Begin in a pike sit, with your hands on the floor behind your hips and your arms slightly bent.

1 Keeping your arms bent, tuck your knees toward your chest.

2 Extend both legs, bending your elbows slightly for balance. Keep your hips on the floor and your knees slightly bent as you extend your legs. Tuck and extend your legs without letting your feet touch the floor.
Repetitions: Do one or two sets of ten tucks.

POSTPARTUM EXERCISES

Exercise No. 21

V-Stretch

1 Open your knees wide, place your toes together, and slide your hands down to your ankles.

2 Pull your feet close to your body, then slowly straighten your legs out to a V position. Hold the position for a few seconds. Do not bounce.

Aim: To tone and strengthen your abdominal muscles, legs, feet, and especially your inner thighs.

Starting Position: Back tuck.

3 Keeping your knees open wide, bring your toes back together, then return to starting position.
Repetitions: Repeat five times.

POSTPARTUM EXERCISES

Exercise No. 22

Leg Raises

Aim: To strengthen your inner and outer thighs, lower back, and buttock muscles.

Starting Position: Lying on your right side with your right knee bent, rest your head on your right arm and steady your body with your left arm.

1 Raise your left leg to a comfortable height, lower it to rest on your right leg. *Repetitions:* Repeat ten times.

2 Raise your left leg slightly and circle it five times forward, then five times backward.

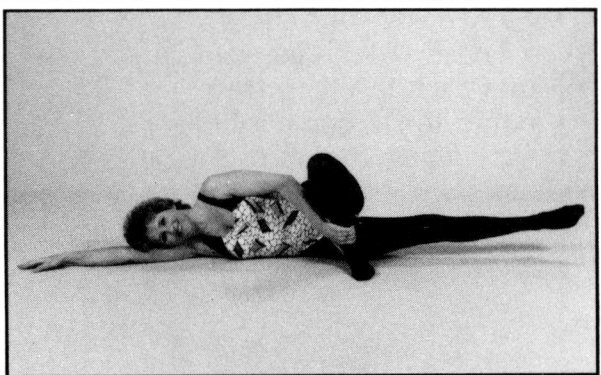

3 Raise your left leg, cross it in front of your right leg, and place it flat on the floor. Point the toes of your right foot, then straighten your right leg and lift it ten times. *Repetitions:* Repeat the entire exercise lying on your left side with your left leg bent.

POSTPARTUM EXERCISES
Exercise No. 23

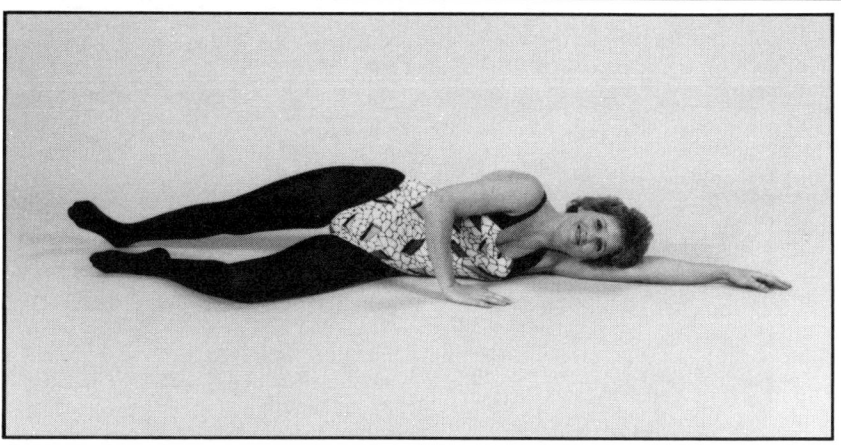

1 Bend your left leg. Raise your right leg five to eight inches off the floor, then touch your right heel down behind your left leg.

2 Bring your right foot to the front and touch your toe to the floor. Do the heel-toe motion five times. Repetitions: Repeat the entire exercise lying on your right side.

Rainbows
(Heel/Toe)

Aim: To tone your hips, legs, waist, and buttocks.

Starting Position: Lying on your left side with your left knee bent, rest your head on your left arm and steady your body with your right arm.

POSTPARTUM EXERCISES

Exercise No. 24

Side Raisers

Aim: To tone your hips, legs, waist, and buttocks.

Starting Position: Lying on your right side with your right knee bent, rest your head on your right arm and steady your body with your left arm.

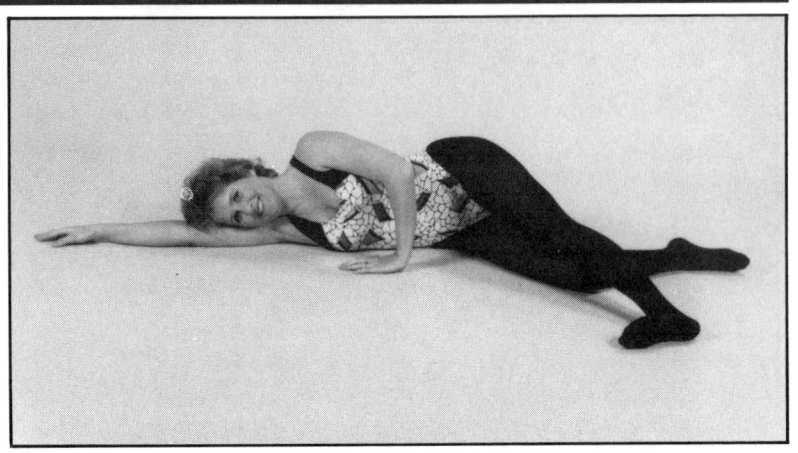

1 Bring your left leg in front of your body to meet your right knee.

2 Extend your left leg with your foot flexed, raise it to hip level, then lower it. Repeat five to ten times, then roll to your left side and repeat the entire exercise.
Repetitions: Repeat five to ten times each side.

POSTPARTUM EXERCISES

Exercise No. 25

Cheek to Cheek

Tighten your buttock muscles. Hold the position for fifteen seconds, then release. *Repetitions:* Repeat three to five times.

Aim: To tone your buttock muscles.

Starting Position: Lying flat on your stomach, with your forehead resting on your folded forearms.

Nursing Variation: Same as above, but lying on your left side.

POSTPARTUM EXERCISES

Exercise No. 26

Leg Circles

Aim: To tone your legs and buttocks.

Starting Position: All fours.

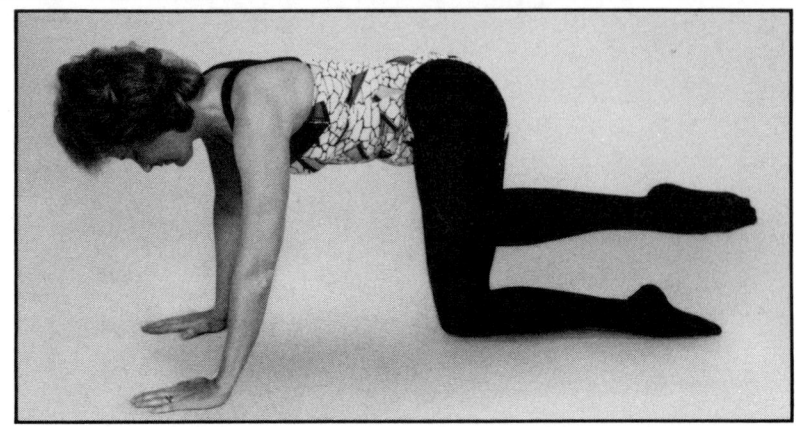

1 Bring your left knee forward toward your chin. Keeping your knees bent, raise your left leg to be parallel to the floor.

2 Keeping your knee parallel to the floor, look straight down at the floor, and circle your leg forward twice with your foot flexed, then twice with your toes pointed.
Repetitions: Repeat on right side. Work up to four sets, alternating sides (twice on each side).

POSTPARTUM EXERCISES

Exercise No. 27

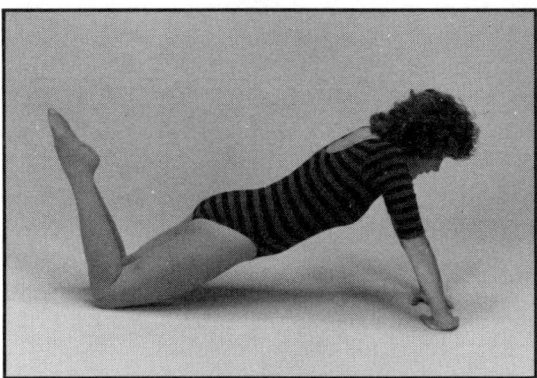

1 Bend your knees and push up, exhaling as you do so.

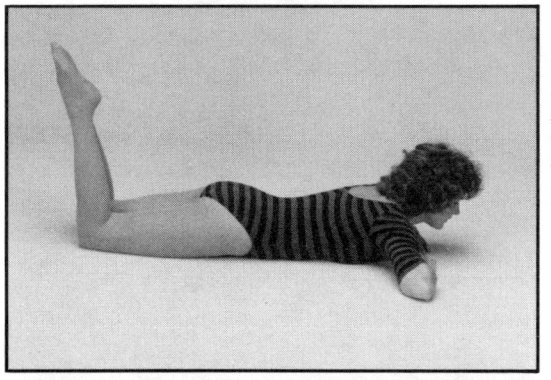

2 Inhale as you slowly lower yourself toward the floor. *Repetitions:* Repeat five times. Add two or three push-ups each week as you gain strength; work up to twenty or more.

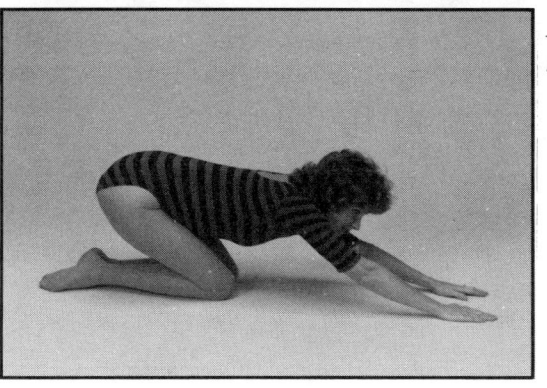

Let-Downs (variation for beginners): Beginning in push-up position with your knees bent (see #1 above), slowly lower your body to the floor. Push your body back so that your hips are aligned with your heels, then return to starting position. *Repetitions:* Repeat three to five times; work up to ten let-downs.

Push-Ups

Aim: To strengthen your shoulders and your pectoral muscles.

Starting Position: Lying flat on your stomach, with your hands under your shoulders and your fingers pointed in.

Note: To make the push-ups more difficult, bring your fingertips closer together. Beginners should start with the *Let-down* variation.

POSTPARTUM EXERCISES

Exercise No. 28

Nursing Exercise

Aim: To loosen up your neck and shoulders and stretch your pectoral muscles.

Starting Position: Tailor sit.

1 Clasp your hands behind your back.

2 Keeping your head centered, lift your arms as you lean forward until you feel a stretch in your pectoral muscles. *Repetitions:* Repeat three to five times.

Note: This is an excellent exercise for nursing moms.

POSTPARTUM EXERCISES

Exercise No. 29

1 Hold onto the outside of your ankle with one hand and cradle your knee with the other arm, as though you were cradling a baby.

Cradle Stretch

2 Slowly pull your right leg toward your chest. Hold the position for fifteen seconds as you circle your right ankle. *Repetitions:* Repeat with your left leg.

Aim: To tone your neck, shoulders, arms, lower back, hips, legs, and buttocks.

Starting Position: Straddle sit, with your toes pointed.

Variation: As you cradle your right knee with your right hand and hold your right calf in your left hand, rock your right leg back and forth and from side to side in a gentle, swaying motion.

POSTPARTUM EXERCISES

Exercise No. 30

Lateral Straddle Stretch

Aim: To strengthen abdominals and hip flexors, and stretch lower back and hamstrings.

Starting Position: Straddle sit, with your toes pointed comfortably and your arms in cross position.

1 Bend your right leg in and bring your left arm forward to the inside of your left leg. Raise your right arm over your head and bend to the left. Repeat five times to the left.

2 Bend forward at the center of your body, holding your chest as close to the floor as possible, and return to straddle sit.

3 Bend your left leg in and bring your right arm forward to the inside of your right leg. Raise your left arm over your head and bend to the right. Repeat five times to the right. Bend forward at the center of your body, holding your chest as close to the floor as possible, and return to straddle sit. *Repetitions:* Repeat the entire exercise once (bending to the left and right five times each).

POSTPARTUM EXERCISES

Exercise No. 30

Lateral Straddle Stretch

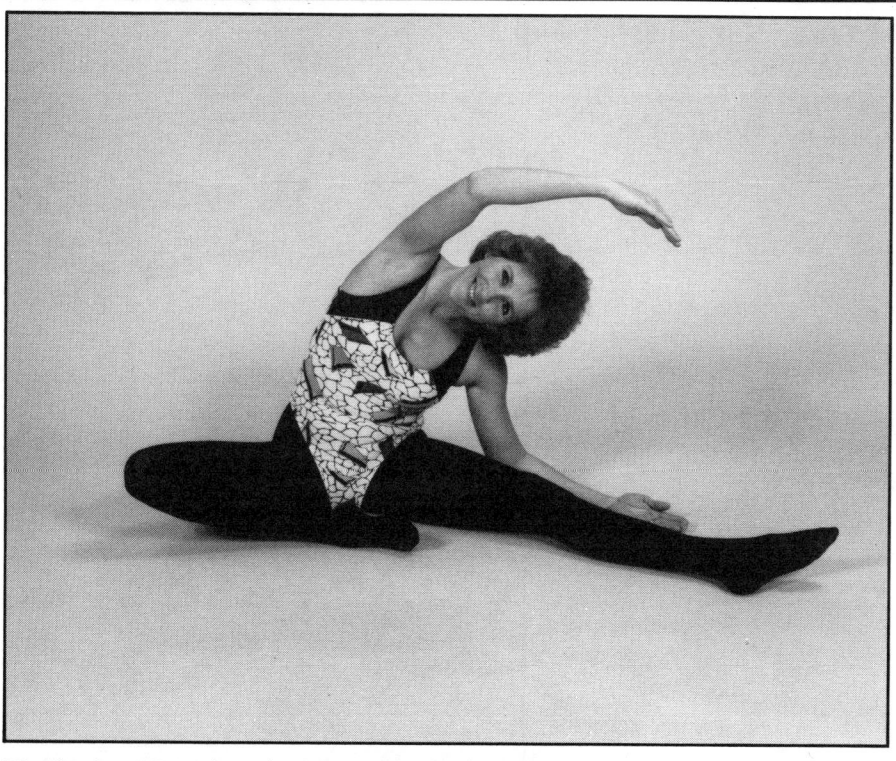

Aim: To strengthen abdominals and hip flexors, and stretch lower back and hamstrings.

Starting Position: Straddle sit, with your toes pointed comfortably and your arms in cross position.

Variation: Bend right leg in and place your left arm on the floor behind your left leg. Bring your right arm over your head and bend to the left. Repeat five times to the left, change legs, and repeat five times to the right.
Repetitions: Repeat the entire exercise once.

POSTPARTUM EXERCISES

Exercise No. 31

Hamstring Straddle Stretch

Aim: To strengthen abdominals and hip flexors, and stretch hamstrings, gluteus, and lower back.

Starting Position: Straddle sit, with your toes pointed comfortably and your arms at your sides.

1 Bend your right leg in, lean left from your hip, and stretch as far forward as you can, looking over your foot. Repeat five times to the left.

2 Bend forward at the center of your body, holding your chest as close to the floor as possible, and return to straddle sit.

3 Bend your left leg in, lean right from your hip, and stretch as far forward as you can, looking over your foot. Repeat five times to the right. Bend forward at the center of your body, holding your chest as close to the floor as possible, and return to straddle sit. *Repetitions:* Repeat the entire exercise once (leaning to the left and right five times each).

POSTPARTUM EXERCISES

Exercise No. 32

Hip Roll

Aim: To trim your hips, waist, and thighs.

Starting Position: Hook-lying, with your arms in cross position.

1 Bring your knees to your chest and roll to the right. Bring your knees back to center, then roll to the left. *Repetitions:* Repeat ten times on each side, alternating sides.

POSTPARTUM EXERCISES

Exercise No. 33

Knee Cross-Overs

Aim: To stretch your lower back muscles and tone your buttock muscles.

Starting Position: Lying on your back with your legs straight out.

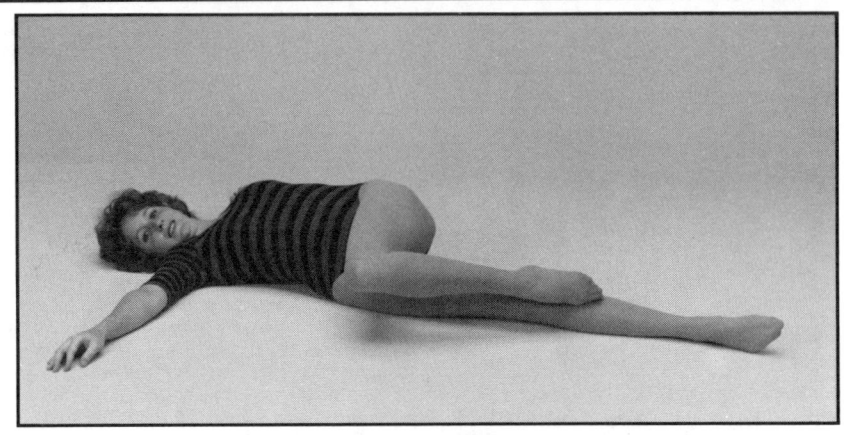

1 Draw your left knee to your chest and cross it over your body. Hold the position for five seconds.

2 Place the instep of your left foot on the inside of your right knee. Hold your left knee as close to the floor as is comfortable, until you feel a stretch. Hold the position for five seconds, then relax. *Repetitions:* Repeat the entire exercise three to five times with each leg, alternating legs.

POSTPARTUM EXERCISES

Exercise No. 34

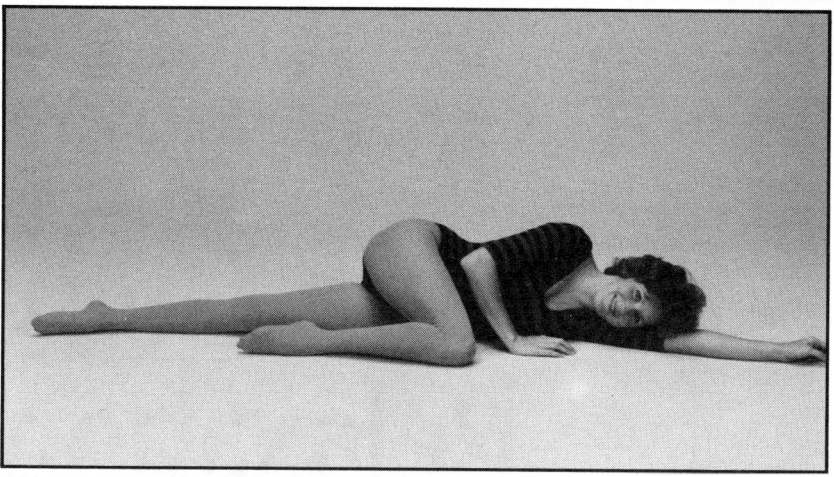

1 Bring your right knee over your left side, shifting your weight to your right hip as you do so.

2 Keeping your right knee on the floor, glide it toward your chest and back down until your leg is almost straight. *Repetitions:* Repeat three times on each side.

Knee Gliders

Aim: To relax your lower back, hips, and buttock muscles.

Starting Position: Lying on your left side with your head resting comfortably on your arm, and with your hips and knees slightly bent.

POSTPARTUM EXERCISES

Exercise No. 35

Body Relaxation

Aim: To relax you.

Starting Position: Lying on your left side.

1 Concentrate on something or somewhere very peaceful. Close your eyes and take deep breaths. In the following order, relax your *feet, legs, back, arms, neck, and face*. After you feel totally relaxed and peaceful, open your eyes, roll to all fours, and slowly stand up.

Chapter Four
Postpartum Strength-training Routine

Let's start with a brief introduction to resistance equipment. Equipment like Nautilus and Universal has revolutionized strength training. You can use these machines to help recover from an injury, train for sports, bodybuild, supplement your aerobic workout, and prevent exercise injuries—with as little as a three-hour-a-week commitment, an hour every other day.

Most machines are designed according to the body's normal range of motion. Ideally, each machine incorporates these ten basic requirements of full-range exercise:*

1. *Positive work*—lifting a weight
2. *Negative work*—lowering a weight
3. *Rotary movement*—rotating the body part as it works around the axis of a joint
4. *Stretching*—exceeding the existing range of movement
5. *Prestretching*—increased tension prior to the start of a contraction
6. *Automatically variable resistance*—the cam changes resistance as movement occurs
7. *Balanced resistance*—resistance according to your strength in each position
8. *Direct resistance*—resistance applied to the body part or muscle being worked
9. *Resistance in position of full muscular contraction*—resistance in the finishing position
10. *Unrestricted speed of movement*—speed should vary during the exercise

To assure that you achieve this full range of motion when you exercise, follow these basic guidelines:

1. Before your first workout, have a trained instructor orient you to the equipment to make sure you learn to use it properly.

2. Be sure your body is positioned correctly in each machine (i.e., add a pad, raise or lower the seat).

3. Perform each exercise (machine) eight to twelve repetitions. *Note:* Have a trained instructor help you find a starting weightload on each machine. If you can do twelve repetitions easily, then it's time to increase your weightload. If you can't do eight repetitions, then you need to decrease your weightload.

4. Breathe normally. Exhale on the lifting and inhale during the lowering (negative resistance). Do not hold your breath while lifting a weight.

5. Move quickly from machine to machine for effective cardiovascular conditioning throughout the routine.

The following routine is designed to tone up your entire body after you have the baby. It includes floor exercises, a stationary bicycle workout, and a resistance equipment workout. Once you start to see the results of muscle toning, you won't want to stop!

Note: As with any exercise routine, check with your physician before you start a strength-training program.

*__Source:__ Dr. Ellington Darden, *New Nautilus Book* (Ellington Darden, Darden Research Corporation, Box 1016, Lake Helen, FL 32744).

POSTPARTUM STRENGTH TRAINING

This routine may be done three different ways:

1. Try this routine as a supplement to the postpartum exercise routine in Chapter 3. For example, do the postpartum exercise routine three days a week (Monday, Wednesday, Friday) and this strength-training routine two days a week (Tuesday and Thursday). This routine allows you a two-day recovery period over the weekend. This, of course, is the ideal program.

2. This routine can be your only workout, but then you need to do it three days a week. It is recommended that you follow an every-other-day format when using resistance equipment, which allows your muscles a day of rest between workouts. You may want to run or swim on this in-between day.

3. The floor exercises can be done alone, especially in the first weeks after the baby is born, to supplement the cesarean hospital exercises (p. 78) or the vaginal hospital exercises (p. 84). After receiving your doctor's okay, add the bicycle and resistance equipment.

Note: Check with your physician on when you can add the floor exercises, especially if you have had a cesarean delivery.

The Routine

1. **Floor Exercises**—Your workout should include these exercises, which begin on page 138:

   1. Lateral Straddle Stretch (page 138) and Variation (page 139)
   2. Hamstring Straddle Stretch (page 140)
   3. Leg Raises (page 141)
   4. Rainbows (page 142)
   5. Curl-Ups (page 143) and Oblique Curl-Ups (page 144)
   6. Push-ups (page 145)
   7. Arm Series (pages 146-147)

2. **Stationary Bicycle**—Do a twelve- to fifteen-minute workout. *Note:* If a stationary bicycle is not available, substitute a bike ride and/or the bicycle exercise on page 113.

3. **Resistance Equipment**—Add Nautilus or Universal machines. Be sure to have a trained instructor locate each machine and show you how to use it.

Most weight rooms are set up in a circuit, with the machines following a particular order. Normally, the machines that exercise the larger muscle groups (lower body) come first; those that exercise the smaller muscle groups (upper body) follow. Also note that some machines do more than one exercise.

To set up your routine, select one exercise/machine for each muscle group. Include four to six machines/exercises for the lower body and six to eight for the upper body, for a total of twelve machines/exercises in your routine. If you have a bad back, use the hip and back machines with caution or avoid them completely. (See the list of machines to use with caution in the strength-training guidelines in Chapter 1, p. 13.)

The following chart lists Nautilus and Universal machines that correspond to the basic muscle groups, as stated in the "Aim." Corresponding floor exercises are included, as well. Also check the "Notes" for any additional guidelines or comments.

To assist you in your workout, prepare a card to record your progress. List the machines included in your workout—in order of completion—on the card. Include with each exercise the correct seat position and whether a pad is needed. Then use the card during every workout to record your weightloads and the repetitions completed.

POSTPARTUM STRENGTH TRAINING

Aim	Floor Exercise	Resistance Equipment		Notes
		Nautilus	**Universal**	
To tone your quadriceps, calves, and gluteus maximus	Lateral Straddle Stretch (pp. 138–139)	Compound Leg Leg Extension Leg Press Calf Raise	Leg Squat Leg Extension Leg Press (includes calf raise)	
To tone your hamstrings and gluteus maximus	Hamstring Straddle Stretch (p. 140)	Leg Curl Duo Hip & Back Duo Squat	Leg Curl Back Hip Extension Leg Press	
To tone your inner/outer thighs and gluteus maximus	Leg Raises (p. 141) Rainbows (p. 142)	Hip Adductor/Abductor	Total Hip	
To strengthen your abdominal muscle (rectus abdominus) and lower back	Curl-Ups (p. 143)	Abdominal Lower Back	Crunch Bench Seated Back	Be sure to check the self-test for separation of the rectus abdominal muscles (see p. 7). If two or more, start with just the floor exercise; then add the machine.
To strengthen your internal and external oblique muscles	Oblique Curl-Ups (p. 144)	Rotary Torso	Rotary Torso	
To strengthen your shoulders, triceps, and pectoral muscles	Push-Ups (p. 145)	Multitricep Overhead Press (Bench Press)	High Pulley Chest Press	
To stretch your pectoral and deltoid (shoulder) muscles	Scissors (p. 146)	Double Chest Women's Chest Chest/Shoulder Lateral Raise	Chest Press Incline Fly Vertical Chest Seated Chest	Pick 1–2 of the machines available in this group.
To strengthen your latissimus dorsi muscles of the back	Elbows Together (p. 146)	Torso Arm Pullover	High Pulley	
To strengthen and tone your upper-arm biceps	Elbow Flex (p. 147)	Multibicep	Arm Curl	
To strengthen your deltoid and trapezius muscles	Arm Circles (forward and backward) (p. 147)	Rowing Torso Double Shoulder	Low Pulley	

POSTPARTUM STRENGTH TRAINING

Exercise No. 1

Lateral Straddle Stretch

Aim: To strengthen abdominals and hip flexors, and stretch lower back and hamstrings.

Starting Position: Straddle sit, with your toes pointed comfortably and your arms in cross position.

1 Bend your right leg in and bring your left arm forward to the inside of your left leg. Raise your right arm over your head and bend to the left. Repeat five times to the left.

2 Bend forward at the center of your body, holding your chest as close to the floor as possible, and return to straddle sit.

3 Bend left leg in and bring right arm forward to the inside of your right leg. Raise your left arm over your head and bend to the right. Repeat five times to the right. Bend forward at the center of your body, holding your chest as close to the floor as possible, and return to straddle sit. *Repetitions:* Repeat the entire exercise once (bending to the left and right five times each).

POSTPARTUM STRENGTH TRAINING

Exercise No. 1

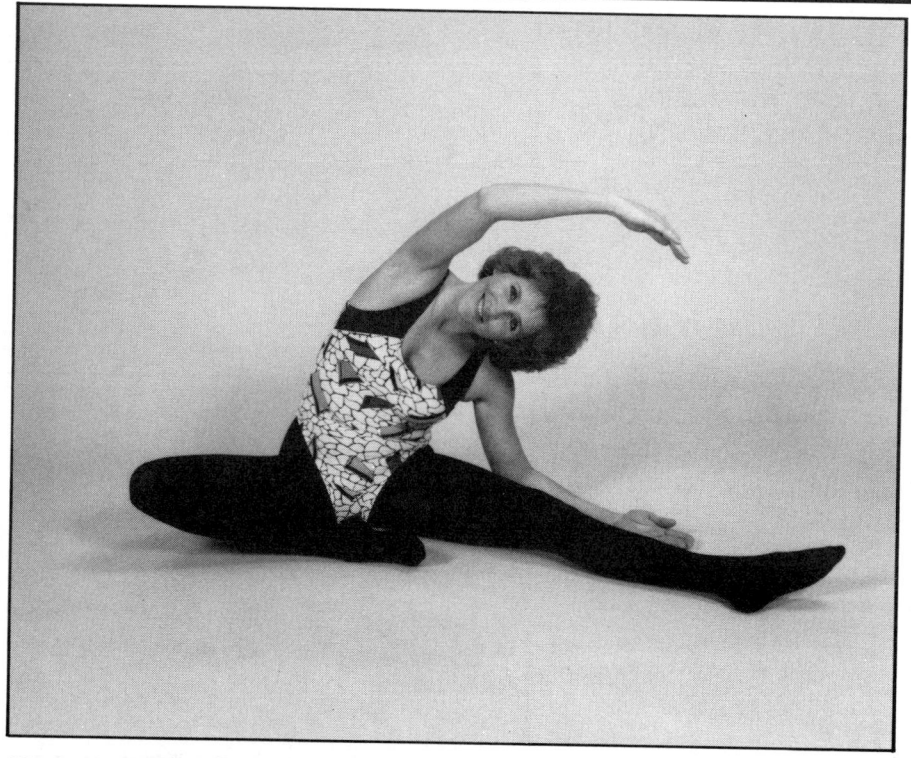

Lateral Straddle Stretch

Aim: To strengthen abdominals and hip flexors, and stretch lower back and hamstrings.

Starting Position: Straddle sit, with your toes pointed comfortably and your arms in cross position.

Variation: Bend right leg in and place your left arm on the floor behind your left leg. Raise your right arm over your head and bend to the left. Repeat five times to the left, change legs, and repeat five times to the right.
Repetitions: Repeat the entire exercise once.

POSTPARTUM STRENGTH TRAINING

Exercise No. 2

Hamstring Straddle Stretch

Aim: To strengthen abdominals and hip flexors, and stretch hamstrings, gluteus, and lower back.

Starting Position: Straddle sit, with your toes pointed comfortably and your arms at your sides.

1 Bend your right leg in, lean left from your hip, and stretch as far forward as you can, looking over your foot. Repeat five times to the left.

2 Bend forward at the center of your body, holding your chest as close to the floor as possible, and return to straddle sit.

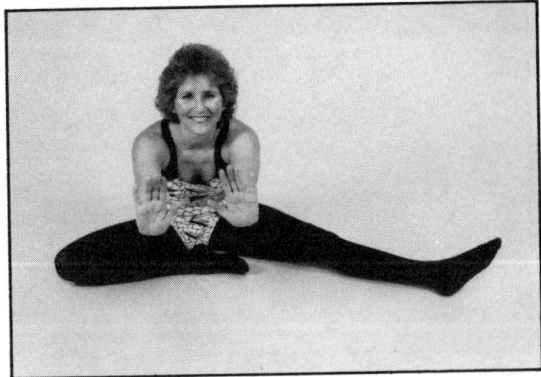

3 Bend your left leg in, lean right from your hip, and stretch as far forward as you can, looking over your foot. Repeat five times to the right. Bend forward at the center of your body, holding your chest as close to the floor as possible, and return to straddle sit. *Repetitions:* Repeat the entire exercise once (leaning to the left and right five times each).

POSTPARTUM STRENGTH TRAINING

Exercise No. 3

Leg Raises

1 Raise your right leg to a comfortable height, then lower it to rest on your left leg. *Repetitions:* Repeat ten times.

2 Raise your right leg slightly and circle it five times forward, then five times backward.

3 Raise your right leg, cross it in front of your left leg, and place it flat on the floor. Point the toes of your left foot, then straighten your left leg and lift it ten times. *Repetitions:* Repeat the entire exercise lying on your right side, with your right leg bent.

Aim: To strengthen your inner and outer thighs, lower back, and buttock muscles.

Starting Position: Lying on your left side with your left knee bent, rest your head on your left arm, and steady your body with your right arm.

POSTPARTUM STRENGTH TRAINING

Exercise No. 4

Rainbows
(Heel/Toe)

Aim: To tone your hips, legs, waist, and buttocks.

Starting Position: Lying on your right side with your right knee bent, rest your head on your right arm, and steady your body with your left arm.

1 Bend your right leg. Raise your left leg five to eight inches off the floor, then touch your left heel down behind your right leg.

2 Bring your left foot to the front and touch your toe to the floor. Do the heel/toe motion five times, then reverse and do a toe/heel motion five times. *Repetitions:* Repeat the entire exercise lying on your left side.

POSTPARTUM STRENGTH TRAINING

Exercise No. 5

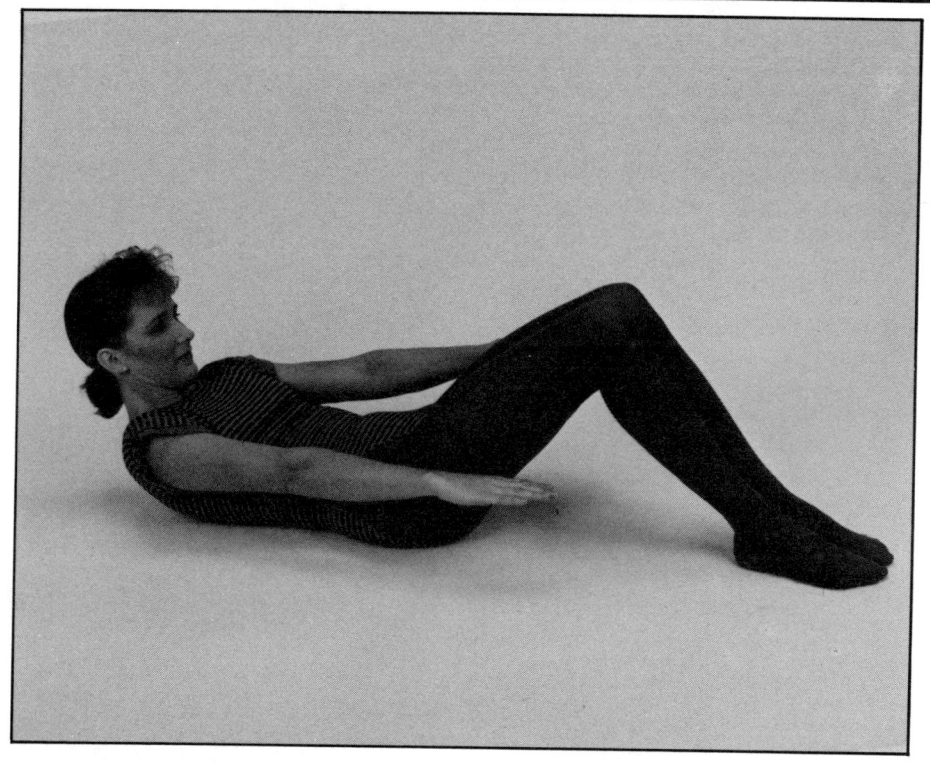

Curl-Ups

Aim: To strengthen your abdominal muscles and lower back.

Starting Positions: #1. Hook-lying, with your arms crossed, holding your ribs. Or #2. Hook-lying, with your arms bent and your fingers locked or hands crossed on top of your head.

Lie on your back, with your knees bent, keeping your feet flat on the floor. Curl up slowly (don't jerk), just far enough for your shoulder blades to come off the floor. Hold your head and neck tight, in a fixed position. Lower to starting position.

Note: Hold your chin to your chest when curling up.
Repetitions: Start with five and work up to thirty or more.

POSTPARTUM STRENGTH TRAINING

Exercise No. 5

Oblique Curl-Ups

Aim: To strengthen your oblique abdominal muscles.

Starting Position: If you have recti diastasis, use starting position #1 on page 143. Otherwise, use starting position #2 on page 143.

1 Curl up, lifting your right shoulder. Point your right elbow toward your left knee, and curl back down. Repeat.

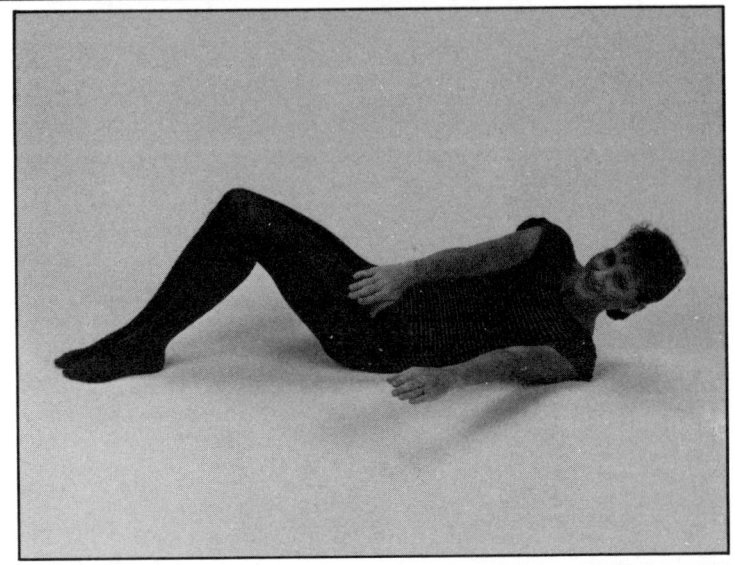

2 Curl up, lifting your left shoulder. Point your left elbow toward your right knee, and curl back down. *Repetitions:* Start with five on each side, alternating, and work up to twenty (ten on each side) or more.

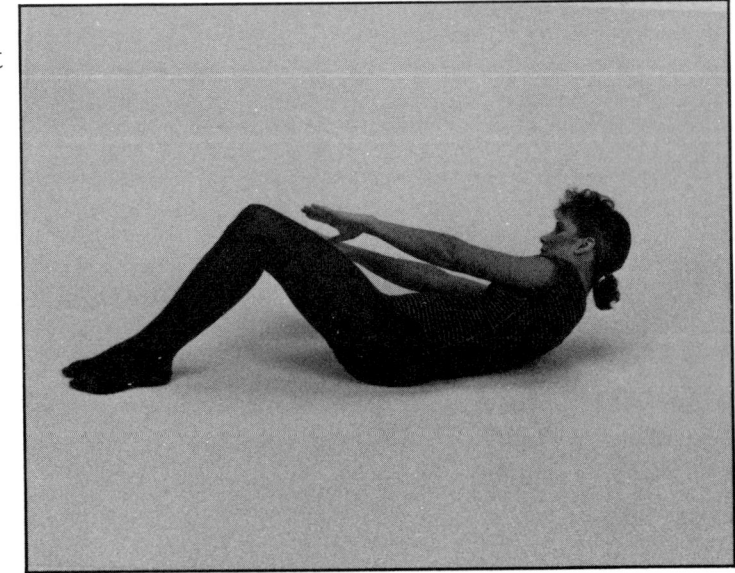

POSTPARTUM STRENGTH TRAINING

Exercise No. 6

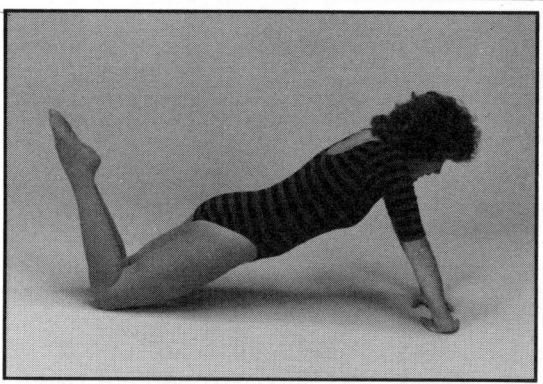

1 Bend your knees and push up, exhaling as you do so.

2 Inhale as you slowly lower yourself toward the floor. *Repetitions:* Repeat five times. Add two or three push-ups each week as you gain strength; work up to twenty or more.

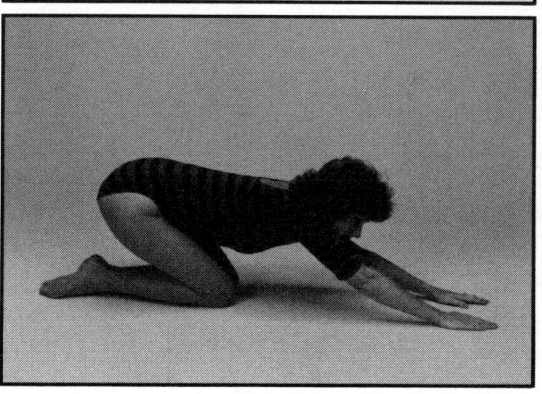

Let-Downs (variation for beginners): Beginning in push-up position with knees bent (see #1 above), slowly lower your body to the floor. Push your body back so that your hips are aligned with your heels, then return to starting position. *Repetitions:* Repeat three to five times; work up to ten let-downs.

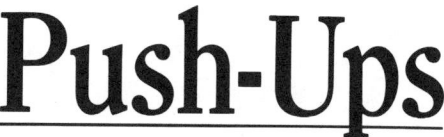

Push-Ups

Aim: To strengthen your shoulders and your pectoral muscles.

Starting Position: Lying flat on your stomach, with your hands under your shoulders and your fingers pointed in.

Note: To make the push-ups more difficult, bring your fingertips closer together. Beginners should start with the *Let-Down* variation.

POSTPARTUM STRENGTH TRAINING

Exercise No. 7

Arm Series

Aim: To strengthen your upper and lower arms, wrists, and pectoral muscles.

Starting Position: Standing, with your feet shoulder-width apart and your arms in cross position.

Scissors: Hold your arms out, straight in front of your body, with your palms down. Move your arms in a scissors motion, alternating right over left arm and left over right arm. *Repetitions:* Repeat the entire exercise with your palms up ten times and with your palms down ten times.

Elbows Together: Bend your arms at the elbows. Tightening your arms, make fists, and bring your forearms together in front of your body. Press your arms open to cross position. *Repetitions:* Repeat five to ten times.

POSTPARTUM STRENGTH TRAINING

Exercise No. 7

1 *Elbow Flex:* With your palms up, make fists.

2 Bend your elbows until your fists touch your shoulders, then circle forearms downward and outward until extended.

3 Turn your fists toward the ceiling.

4 Bend your elbows and touch your fists to your shoulders, then return to starting position.
Repetitions: Repeat entire exercise five times.

Arm Series

Aim: To strengthen your upper and lower arms, wrists, and pectoral muscles.

Starting Position: Standing, with your feet shoulderwidth apart and your arms in cross position.

POSTPARTUM STRENGTH TRAINING

Exercise No. 7

Arm Series

Aim: To strengthen your upper and lower arms, wrists, and pectoral muscles.

Starting Position: Standing, with your feet shoulder width apart and your arms in a cross position.

1 With your palms up, move your arms forward to make five to ten small circles.

2 With your palms up, move your arms forward to make five to ten large circles. *Repetitions:* Repeat, moving your arms backward, then repeat with your palms down.

Chapter Five
Focus on the Baby

Baby exercises? Yes! You can begin exercising with your baby right from the start. This chapter includes a section on massages for your baby, a description of your baby's reflexes that can be "patterned" through exercise to help your baby develop coordination and motor skills, and two sets of parent/baby exercises—one for newborn to four-month-old babies, the other for four- to twelve-month-old babies. At the end of this chapter are directions for making your own exercise equipment (an exercise mat/roll and a beanbag chair).

These parent/baby exercises give you a time to play meaningfully with your child and encourage self-discovery and the development of physical control in your baby. These activities also begin to establish movement patterns, stimulate your baby's circulation, and help his or her muscular development. In addition, parent/baby exercise helps your child become aware early on that daily exercise is a vital part of health.

These exercises follow the natural sequence of motor skill development, providing the fundamentals for sitting, crawling, and walking. While there is no guarantee that a child who does the exercises will walk earlier or recognize you sooner than a child who does not, the exercises will help you guide and encourage your child's motor development.

Suggestions for Exercising Your Baby

When should you exercise your baby? With babies, it is not important that you set aside a certain time of day to do an exercise routine. Rather, you should fit the exercise techniques into your baby's everyday activities. For example:

• Start the baby's day with a stimulating massage, followed by some stretching exercises.

• After a bath or prior to naptime, try one of the relaxation exercises or relaxing massages.

• After naptime, work on patterning and exercises related to developing the baby's motor skills.

• Before bedtime, practice relaxation exercises, followed by a relaxing massage.

For older babies, continue to use massage or relaxation techniques that include a range of motion for the joints. Add two or three exercises at a time, depending on your baby's muscle strength and motor skill level. The Family Team Exercises on pages 184 to 198 will provide exercise both for you and your baby. There are even some exercises for mom, dad, and baby to do as a family.

> • Exercise on a soft, warm, secure surface.
> • Make your baby feel secure by supporting him or her properly.
> • Don't overtire your baby. A reasonable amount of time for a newborn is five minutes.
> • Don't ever strain or put pressure on the baby.
> • Don't exercise body joints after eating.
> • Exercise with your baby for short periods of time, several times a day.
> • Increase the length of exercise time as the baby gets older.
> • Always move body parts through natural motions (i.e., no side movement of knees).
> • Relax and have fun. Exercise is a time to be enjoyed by both parents and child.

Do's and Don'ts for Exercising Your Baby

BABY MASSAGE

Baby Massage

Massage provides a unique way to relate to your baby, while offering him a number of benefits: it maintains his levels of activity and movement, stimulates his sense of touch, helps him relax, tones his muscles, and can stimulate his organic and psychological growth. At the same time, massage enhances your feelings of competence in being able to handle your child. Most of all, baby massage gives you a special time together each day. Practice the three massages to help you get started with a regular baby massage routine.

Basic Directions

- Choose a warm place (e.g., the side of a pool or a bathtub) for a massage, and be sure your hands are warm.

- Use firm but gentle strokes.

- Maintain hand and eye contact with your baby throughout the massage, and don't lift your hands off and on the baby.

- Talk to your baby. Let your touch tell him how much you love him.

Vocabulary

Milk—with a light squeeze, move your hands "toward the heart" for circulation benefits. Work on one area at a time—for example, when massaging the baby's arm, milk from his hand to his shoulder. For a relaxing massage, milk "outward from the heat," i.e., move from the warmer to cooler areas of the body.

Comb—with your hand open and fingers spread, try for a lighter touch with each combing action (watch your nails to avoid scratching the baby).

Rake—a milking motion, using alternate sides of your hands.

Stimulating Massage

Note: This massage is best used prior to exercising. Don't do it right before nap- or bedtime, as it will tend to stimulate your baby.

Starting Position: Lay your baby on her back on a firm, comfortable surface.

1. Using a small circular motion, massage, in the following order: a) her stomach; b) her chest; c) her shoulders; d) the back of her neck; e) the back of her head; f) the top of her head; g) her temples.

BABY MASSAGE

2 Using a slight sweeping motion with your thumb, massage: a) her forehead, from center to hairline; b) around her eyes—circle one way, then the other; c) the sides of her nose—sweep down and across to her cheeks; d) her cheeks—stroke from her chin diagonally to her hairline; e) her mouth—circle your finger around her lips one way, then the other; f) her chin—circle your finger around her chin one way, then the other.

5 Using a circular motion, massage your baby's trunk down her left leg, then: a) using a milking stroke, massage her left leg; b) flex her left hip and circle it in a range of motion; c) flex her left knee and rotate her hip in and out.

3 Using small, circular motions, massage her chest; then rake her abdominal area.

6 Circle her left ankle and separate her toes. Then, using your thumbs, massage the sole of her left foot from heel to toes. Shake her left foot and squeeze it gently. Repeat steps 5 and 6 with her right leg.

4 Massage her left arm, then: a) stroke the back of her left hand and palm, then separate her fingers; b) gently shake and squeeze her left hand; c) using a range of motion, bend her left elbow, straighten it, then circle her left arm, rotating it in and out; d) milk her left arm gently and massage her chest. Repeat step 4 with her right arm.

7 Turn your baby onto her stomach (if she won't lie on her stomach, try placing her stomach across your legs), then: a) using your cupped hand, massage your baby starting at her neck, then moving your hand down to her buttocks, and then to her heel; b) comb her back with your fingers (watch out for your fingernails).

BABY MASSAGE

Relaxing Massage

Note: Best used prior to bedtime or naptime, or with a fussy baby.

Starting Position: Lay your baby on his back or across your lap.

1 Using small, circular motions with your fingers, massage around your baby's face and head, over his shoulders, and on his chest.

2 Milk his left arm outward, then shake and gently squeeze his left hand. Repeat with his right arm.

3 Using small, circular motions with your fingers, massage your baby's trunk down his left leg. Then: a) roll his left leg between your hands; and b) with your thumbs, massage the sole of his left foot from heel to toes. Repeat steps with his right leg. Shake the baby's legs, then comb his chest and squeeze each of his feet twice.

Simple Back Massage

Starting Position: Lay your baby face down on a soft towel or on your lap.

1 Using small, circular motions, massage your baby, starting at the back of her neck. a) Go down her shoulders to her arms, then squeeze her hands gently; b) go down her back, buttocks, and legs; c) gently squeeze her calves and feet; d) go up her legs, buttocks, and back to the back of her neck; e) comb her back.

PATTERNING YOUR BABY'S REFLEXES

Patterning Your Baby's Reflexes

Infants can make very few voluntary movements other than a few with their arms and legs. Most of the movements they do make are reflexive—i.e., automatic reactions to stimulation. As infants repeat these movements over and over, they begin to develop patterns that become the basis for voluntary movements later. Stimulating these movements through the use of exercises you can do with your baby can help him or her develop appropriate patterns.

This type of patterning can be done with babies in a way that allows a joint to move through a specific range of movement while coordinating with the movement of another joint. While this process does not assure earlier completion of any specific motor skill such as crawling or walking, it may aid your baby when his or her perception and physical maturity are developed.

"Patterning" exercises can be used from birth. Chart 4a lists six common reflexes of newborns and four voluntary reflexes that appear later, together with exercises that test the reflexes.

Chart 4a. Exercises for Patterning Your Baby's Reflexes

Name of Reflex	Description	Exercise(s)
1. Stepping	If your baby is placed in a standing position on his feet, he will respond by stepping.	
2. Palmar grasp	Your baby's hand will curl tightly around any object placed in it.	Baby Pull-ups, page 162.
3. Babinski reflex	If you stroke the sole of your baby's foot, her toes will fan out and her big toe will extend.	Relaxation and Foot Toner, page 154.
4. Righting reflex (China doll reflex)	If you hold your baby upright, he will try to keep his head up and his eyes open.	Neck Strength Test, page 167.
5. Tonic neck reflex (fencer position)	When a baby turns her head to one side, with one arm at her side, and extends that arm, the opposite arm flexes. This reflex may help her use the sides of her body separately.	Roll to Side, page 165.
6. Swimming reflex	When a baby is placed in water, he makes swimming motions.	Frog Kick and Whip Kick, page 161.
7. Reciprocal kicking	If you hold your baby straight out in front of you, she will kick her legs alternately. This reflex usually disappears after the first month.	Bicycles, Bicycle Flutters, and Bicycle Scissors, page 163.
8. Neck righting	If your baby's head is turned, his body will follow. This reflex appears when the tonic neck reflex disappears.	Rock 'n' Roll, page 166.
9. Parachute reflex (supporting reflex)	If your baby begins to fall forward from an upright position, she will try to catch herself.	Games on the Roll, pages 178-179.
10. Landau reflex	If a baby is held under his stomach only, he will extend his arms and legs. This reflex indicates back strength.	Sky Diver/Parachute, page 186.

PARENT/BABY EXERCISES (for babies 0-4 months old)

Exercise No. 1

Relaxation

Aim: To relax your baby's body and tone his feet.
Starting Position: Lay your baby on his back.

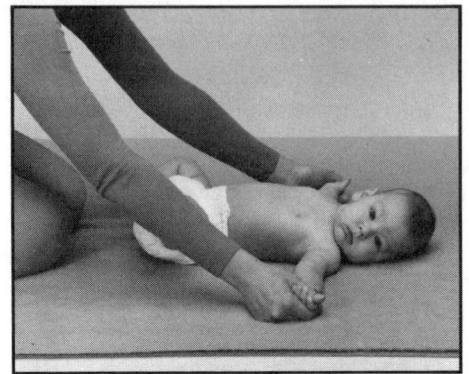

1 Bring his hands together, then slowly lower his arms to cross position.

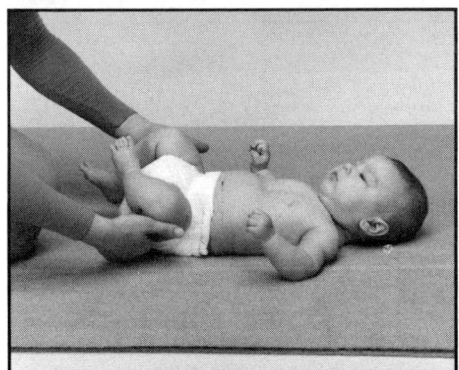

2 Place an index finger under each knee and toss his legs up and down lightly, then bring his knees close to his chest, one at a time. Move his knees only as far as they can easily go—never push or force them.

Foot Toner: Place a finger in the instep of your baby's left foot and place your thumb on the ball of his left foot. Flex his foot, pointing his toes ten times slowly. Circle his foot ten times slowly to the left, then ten times slowly to the right. *Repetitions:* Repeat with his right foot.

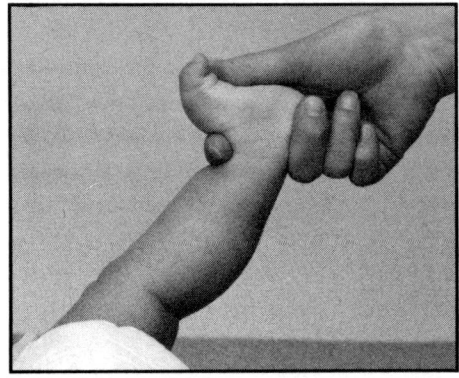

PARENT/BABY EXERCISES (for babies 0-4 months old)

Exercise No. 2

Diaper Change

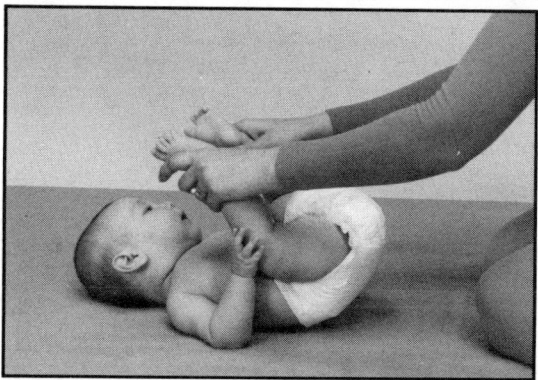

1 Holding your baby's ankles, slowly bring her feet over her head toward the floor. Allow her legs to come back down slowly.
Repetitions: Repeat five times.

1 *Variation:* With your baby in the same starting position, raise her right foot toward her shoulder. Repeat five times on each side, alternating sides.

Aim: To promote flexibility in your baby's back and help relieve gas (especially helpful with colicky babies).

Starting Position: Lay your baby on her back.

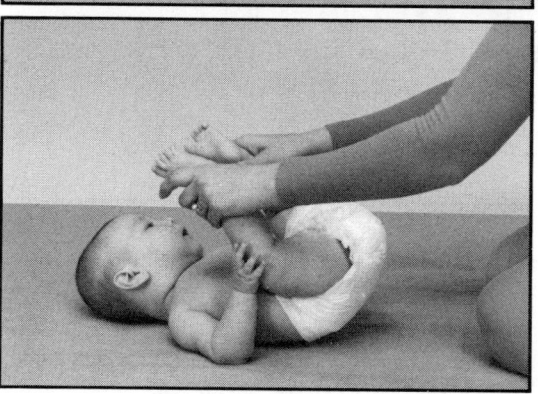

2 Bring both feet over the top of her head and hold for two seconds, then return to starting position.
Repetitions: Repeat once.

Note: Make a game of this exercise by peeking through your baby's legs while they are over her head.

PARENT/BABY EXERCISES (for babies 0-4 months old)

Exercise No. 3

Hug and Rock

Aim: Stretches your baby's arms and promotes his body awareness; may help calm a crying baby.

Starting Position: Lay your baby on his back and cross his arms over his abdomen.

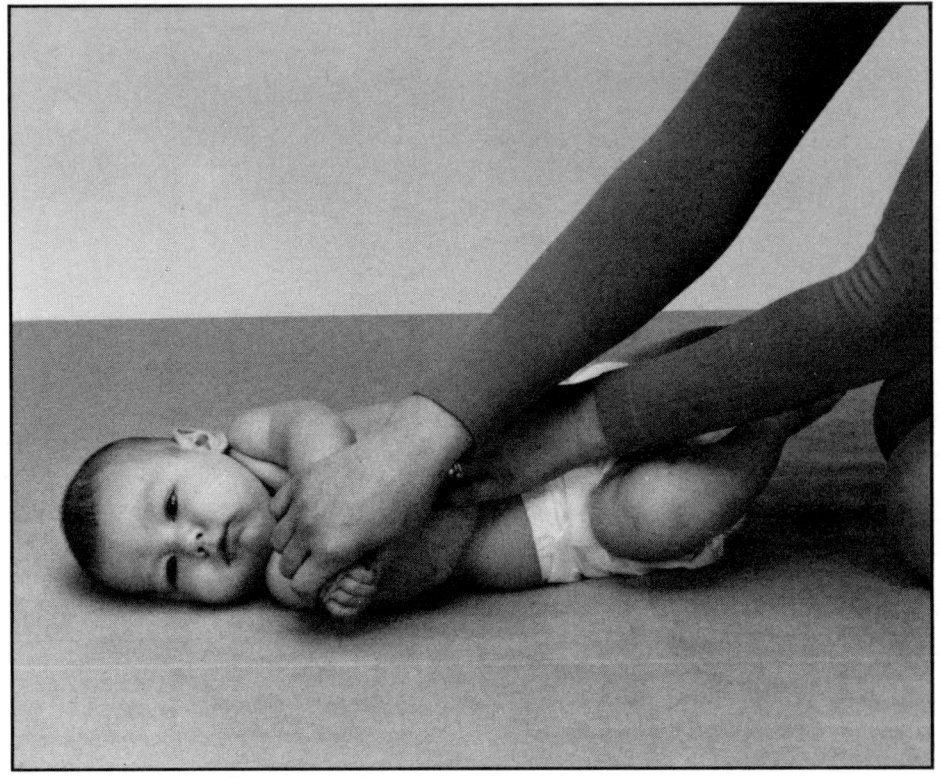

1 Grip your baby's forearms and let him hug himself and touch the rest of his body. Rock him gently to the right and left.

Arm Stretching

EXERCISES (for babies 0-4 months old)

Exercise No. 4

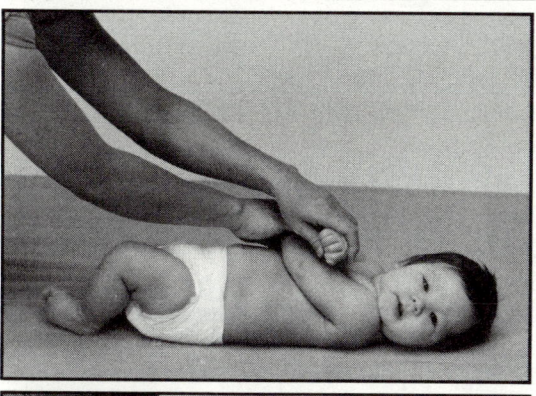

1 Hold [obscured] hand [obscured] arm ove[obscured] then cr[obscured] over he[obscured] *tions:* R[obscured] times w[obscured] nating a[obscured]

2 Raise her left arm above her head, then lower it. Raise her right arm above her head and lower it. *Repetitions:* Repeat three to five times with each arm, alternating arms.

3 Holding your baby's wrists, slowly stretch her arms in a V above her head, then lower her arms.

Aim: To stretch your baby's arms; a good warm-up exercise.

Starting Position: Lay your baby on her back.

Note: To promote your baby's self-esteem, say "yeah" each time you stretch her limbs in the V position, and clap when you finish the exercise.

PARENT/BABY EXERCISES (for babies 0-4 months old)

Exercise No. 4

Leg Stretching

Aim: To stretch your baby's legs; a good warm-up exercise.

Starting Position: Lay your baby on her back.

1 Holding your baby's ankles, cross her left leg over her right leg, then cross her right leg over her left leg. *Repetitions:* Repeat three to five times with each leg, alternating legs.

2 Raise her left leg above her head, then lower it. Raise her right leg above her head, then lower it. *Repetitions:* Repeat three to five times with each leg, alternating legs.

3 Holding onto your baby's ankles, slowly stretch her legs into a V position.

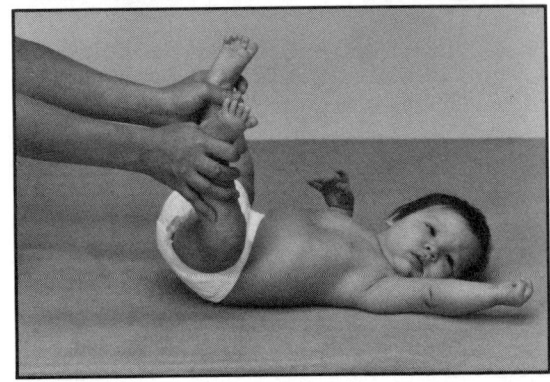

PARENT/BABY EXERCISES (for babies 0-4 months old)

Exercise No. 5

Flex and Extend

1 Bend your baby's knees, bringing them up to his chest.

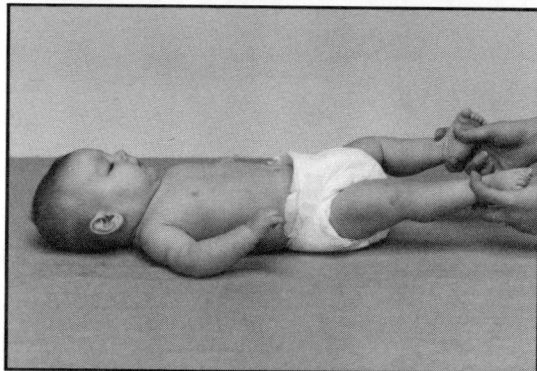

2 Slowly straighten his legs. Be sure your baby's legs are off the floor slightly; never straighten his legs and press them flat to the ground. *Repetitions:* Repeat three to five times.

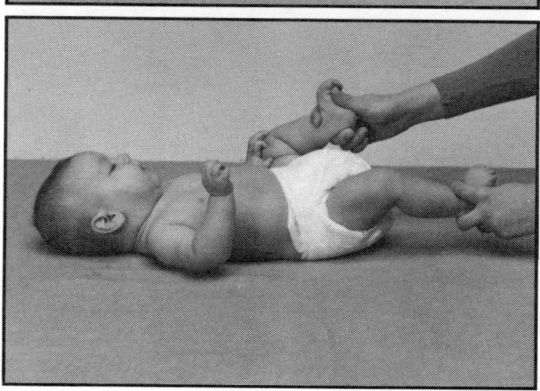

Variation: Alternate bringing his left and right knees to his chest five times.

Aim: To strengthen your baby's thigh muscles and help relieve gas pains.

Starting Position: Lay your baby on his back and hold onto his ankles.

Note: If your baby resists, squeeze his feet and encourage him to relax.

PARENT/BABY EXERCISES (for babies 0-4 months old)

Exercise No. 6

Criss-Cross

Aim: To stretch your baby's arms, legs, and back.

Starting Position: Lay your baby on her back and hold onto her right wrist and left ankle.

1 Cross your baby's right arm and left leg at her middle.

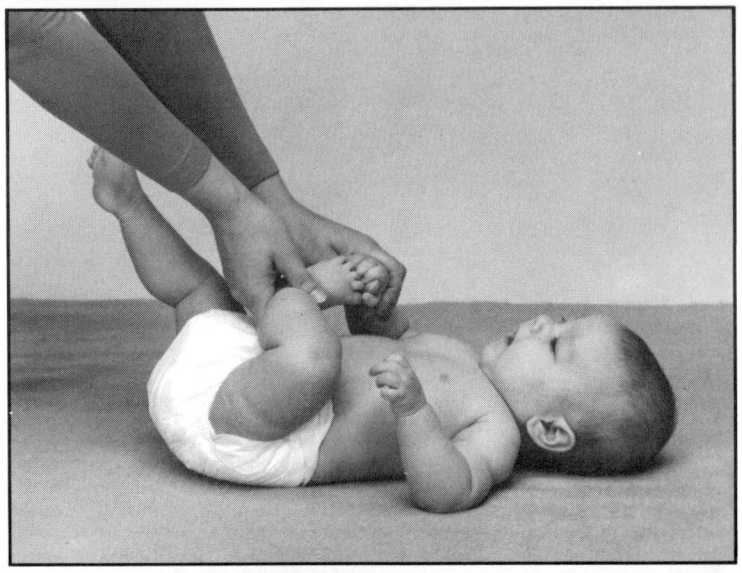

2 Stretch her limbs in opposite directions, then return to starting position. Cross and stretch her left arm and right leg. *Repetitions:* Repeat three to five times on each side, alternating sides.

PARENT/BABY EXERCISES (for babies 0-4 months old)

Exercise No. 7

1 *Frog Kick:* Holding onto your baby's ankles, bend his knees to his chest.

Kicks

2 With his legs slightly off the floor, straighten his legs into a V, then bring his legs back together and bend his knees to his chest. *Repetitions:* Repeat five times.

Aim: To tone your baby's leg muscles.

Starting Position: *Frog Kick:* Lay your baby on his back. *Whip Kick:* Lay your baby on his stomach.

Whip Kick: Hold your baby's ankles and bend his knees. Assist him to kick his seat with his ankles, and extend his legs out, around, and back to starting position. *Repetitions:* Repeat five times.

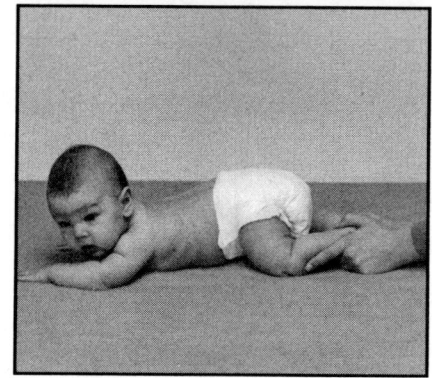

PARENT/BABY EXERCISES (for babies 0-4 months old)

Exercise No. 8

Pull-Ups

Aim: To strengthen your baby's chest, hands and arms.

Starting Position: *Monkey Grip* and *Pull-ups:* Lay your baby on her back. *See-saws:* Pike sit.

1 *Monkey Grip:* Have your baby grasp your thumbs with both hands (Palmar grasp); wrap your index finger around her hands to be sure she holds her grip.

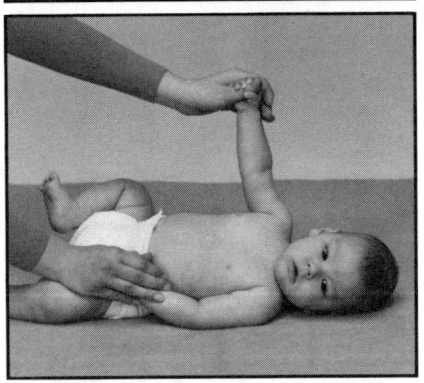

2 Gently pull one arm at a time in an easy upward motion. Do not lift her from the surface, although one shoulder may rise slightly. *Repetitions:* Repeat two or three times with each arm.

Pull-Ups: Repeat step 1 above, then gently pull *both* arms upward until she just begins to lift off the floor. Keeping your hands very still, allow your baby to pull herself up to your fingers. *Repetitions:* Repeat two or three times.

See-Saws (sit-ups for babies two to four months old): Bend your knees and place your baby on your stomach with her facing you, her back against your thighs. Hold her hands as you do sit-ups with her resting on your thighs. *Repetitions:* Repeat five to ten times.

PARENT/BABY EXERCISES (for babies 0-4 months old)

Exercise No. 9

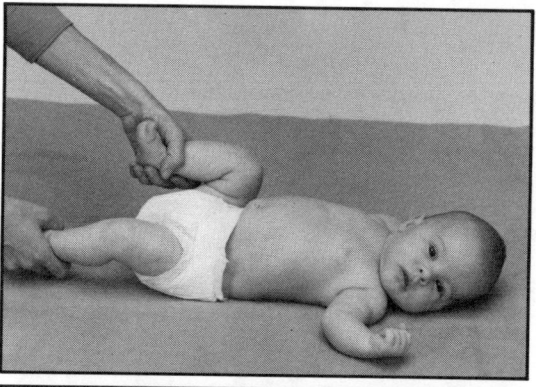

Pedals: Grasp his ankles and pedal his legs in an up-and-down motion for twenty seconds. Lift his hips off the floor slightly and pedal his legs for another twenty seconds.

Bicycles

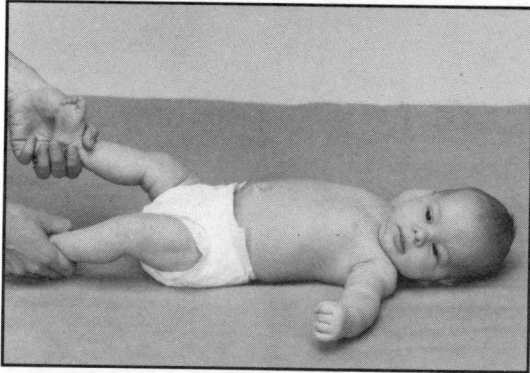

Flutters: Holding onto his feet, extend his legs and lift them off the floor slightly. Make small, light kicking movements (flutters) with the baby's feet for twenty seconds.

Aim: To improve your baby's circulation and exercise his legs at the hip socket.

Starting Position: Lay your baby on his back.

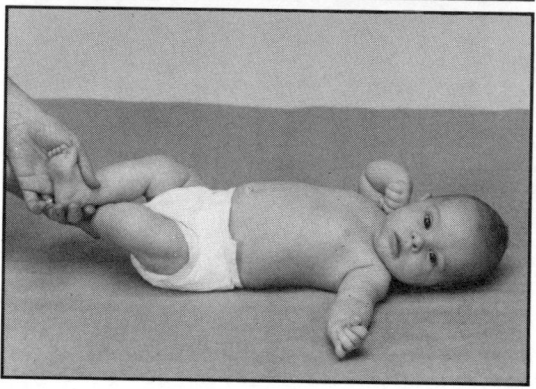

Scissors: Holding his legs straight out in front of him, parallel to the floor, scissor his left leg past his right leg so that his legs just touch. Scissor his right leg past his left leg. *Repetitions:* Repeat ten times, alternating legs.

Note: Never force or push your baby's movements.

PARENT/BABY EXERCISES (for babies 0-4 months old)

Exercise No. 10

Neck Strengtheners

Aim: To strengthen your baby's neck in preparation for crawling.

Starting Position: *Find Me:* Lay your baby on her stomach, with her face turned to her right side. *Look at Me* and *Raising Up:* Sit on the floor and lay your baby on her stomach, with her head resting against your chest.

Note: Before doing *Look at Me*, your baby must be able to turn her head. Before doing *Raising Up*, your baby should be able to lift her head or hold it up. As she gets better at *Raising Up*, have her lie on the towel on an exercise mat instead of on your chest.

Find Me: Go to your baby's left side and call her name. When she moves her head to her left side, smile at her or hand her a favorite toy. Go to her right side and call her name. *Repetitions:* Repeat *no more than* two times to each side.

Look at Me: Lean back until you are resting on your elbows. Talk to your baby; she will lift her head. Do not make her hold her head up longer than ten seconds; then let her rest. Increase the duration as your baby's neck gets stronger.

Raising Up: Same as *Look at Me,* but place a rolled-up towel under your baby's stomach and chest. *Repetitions:* Let your baby hold her head up no longer than ten seconds to start.

PARENT/BABY EXERCISES (for babies 0-4 months old)

Exercise No. 11

Roll to Side

1 Raise your baby's right arm alongside his head. Hold him under his left knee, bend his knee toward his chest, and lift his seat slightly.

2 Roll him slowly onto his right side. *Repetitions:* Repeat, rolling him to his left side, holding his left knee.

Aim: To prepare your baby to roll over.

Starting Position: Lay your baby on his back and place a toy about six inches away from his head.

Note: You can practice this exercise twice a day, but no more than three or four times per session.

PARENT/BABY EXERCISES (for babies 0-4 months old)

Exercise No. 12

Rock 'n' Roll

Aim: To teach your baby to roll from his back to his stomach.

Starting Position: Lay your baby on her back.

1 Bend your baby's left arm and place it on her chest. Flex her right hip, then roll her body to the left.

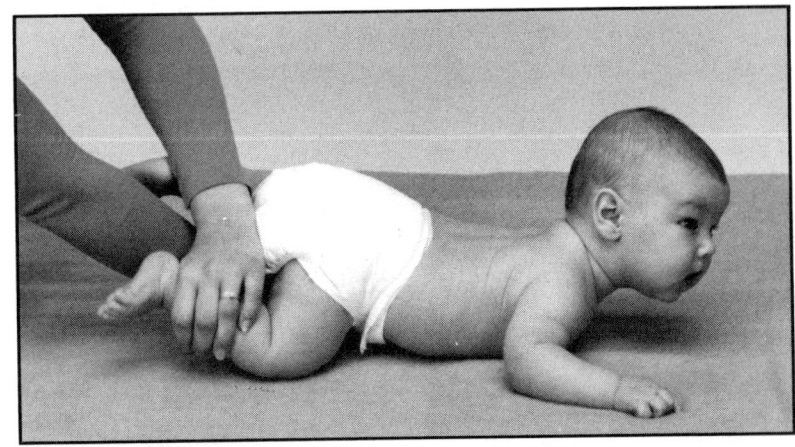

2 She will end up on her stomach. Allow her to try to free her arm, but help her if it appears to be too much of a struggle. *Repetitions:* Repeat two times to the left, then place her right arm across her chest and repeat two times to the right.

Note: Before attempting this exercise, be sure your baby has mastered rolling to her side.

PARENT/BABY EXERCISES (for babies 4-12 months old)

Exercise No. 13

Exercises 13 through 25 (pages 167 to 183) are for babies between four and twelve months old. For exercises that benefit both you and your baby, see the Family Team Exercises on pages 184 to 198.

Strength Test

1. Place one arm across your baby's chest, and the other across his hips.

2. Slide your arm down from his chest, then look to see whether his head drops. If he is not holding his head up, wait two or three weeks before trying the exercises that follow; work on exercise #10, *Neck Strengtheners* (page 164).

Aim: To test your baby's neck muscles to see if he is ready for some of the exercises that follow.

Starting Position: Stand, holding your baby with his back against your chest.

Note: Use this exercise to determine whether or not you should proceed with exercises that require your baby to hold his head up.

PARENT/BABY EXERCISES (for babies 4-12 months old)

Exercise No. 14

Flagpole

Aim: To strengthen your baby's lower back.

Starting Position: Stand, holding your baby with her back against your chest, with your arm across her pelvic area.

Note: Use the *Strength Test* on page 167 to see whether your baby is ready for this exercise.

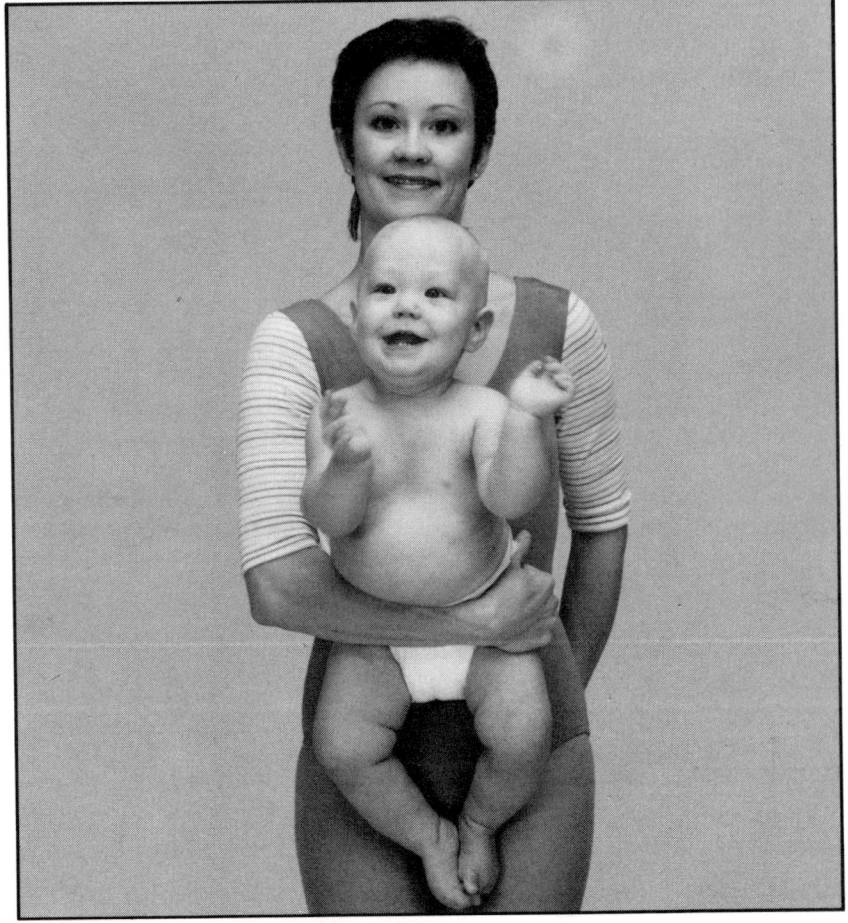

Your baby's hips should be pressed into your abdomen. Hold this position for a few seconds. Practice carrying your baby around the house in this position. In this carrying position, the baby's weight is at your midline, which is good for your posture; and she can see out windows and look in mirrors.

PARENT/BABY EXERCISES (for babies 4-12 months old)

Exercise No. 15

Back Arch

Aim: To strengthen your baby's abdominal muscles.

Starting Position: Pike sit. Lay your baby on his back on your lap, with his head pointing toward your feet.

1 Gently raise your knees so that your baby's back arches slightly. Move slowly and don't raise your knees too high.

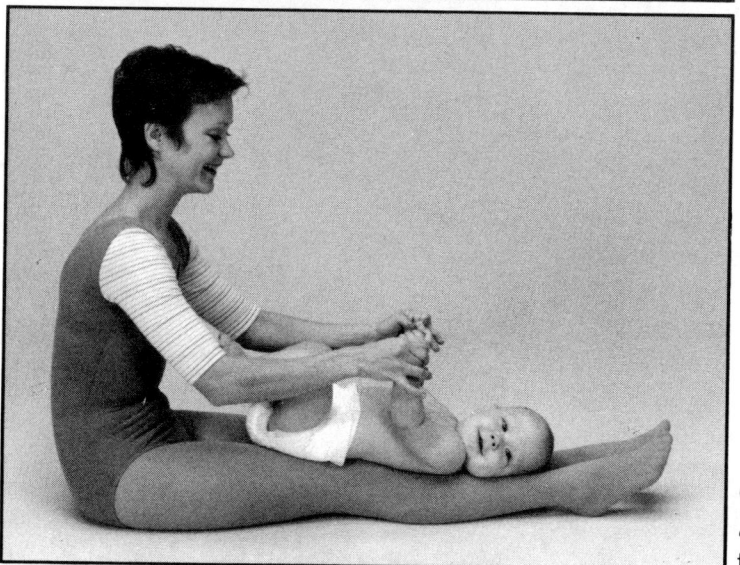

2 Return to starting position. *Repetitions:* Repeat three to five times.

PARENT/BABY EXERCISES (for babies 4-12 months old)

Exercise No. 16

Diaper Change

Aim: To promote flexibility in your baby's back and help relieve gas (especially helpful with colicky babies).

Starting Position: Lay your baby on her back.

1 Holding your baby's ankles, slowly bring her feet over her head toward the floor. Allow her legs to come back down slowly.
Repetitions: Repeat five times.

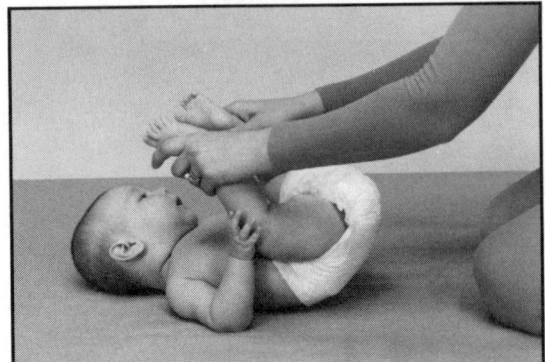

1 *Variation:* With your baby in the same starting position, raise her right foot toward her shoulder. Repeat five times on each side, alternating sides.

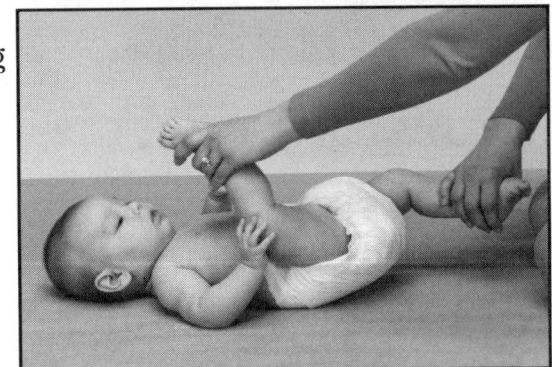

2 Bring both feet over the top of her head and hold for two seconds, then return to starting position.
Repetitions: Repeat once.

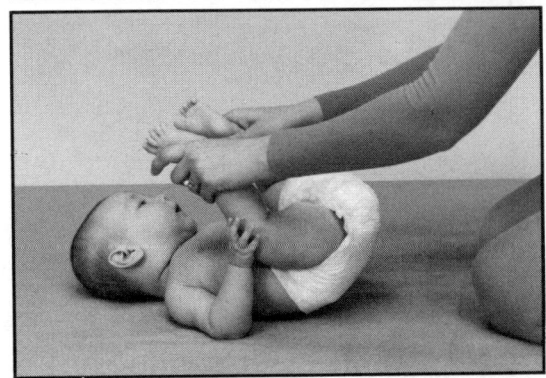

Note: Make a game of this exercise by peeking through your baby's legs while they are over her head.

PARENT/BABY EXERCISES (for babies 4-12 months old)

Exercise No. 17

Arm Stretching

Aim: To stretch your baby's arms and shoulders; a good warm-up exercise.

Starting Position: Lay your baby on his back.

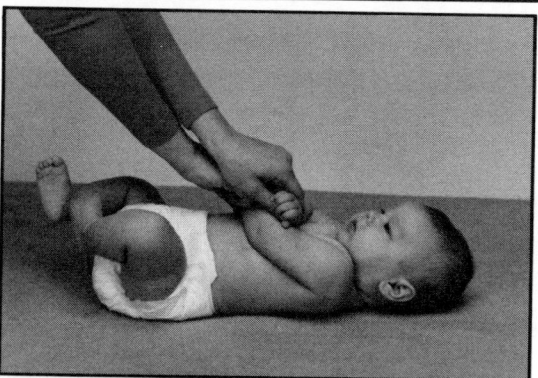

1 Holding your baby's hands, cross his left arm over his right arm, then cross his right arm over his left arm. *Repetitions:* Repeat three to five times with each arm, alternating arms.

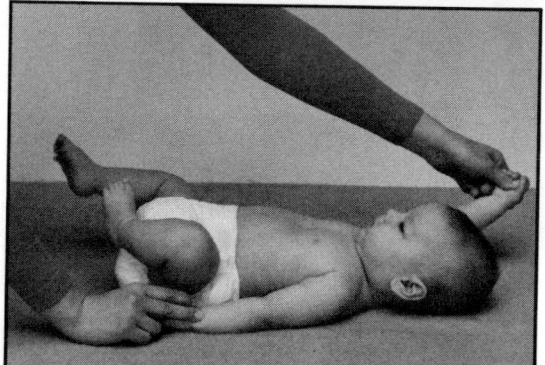

2 Raise his left arm above his head, then lower it to his side. Raise his right arm above his head, then lower it to his side. *Repetitions:* Repeat three to five times with each arm, alternating arms.

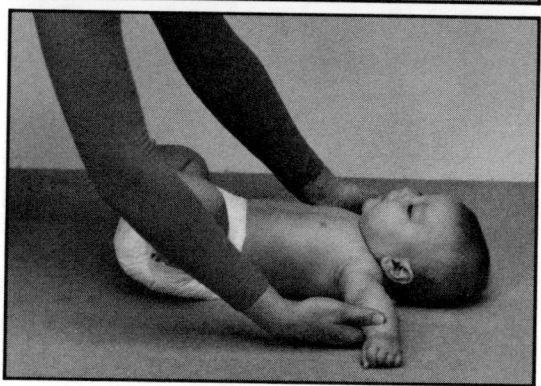

Shoulder Rotations: With your baby's arms at his sides and his palms facing up, hold his upper arms just above his elbows, then gently roll his arms until the palms of his hands are on the floor. Roll his hands back to starting position with palms up. *Repetitions:* Repeat five times slowly.

PARENT/BABY EXERCISES (for babies 4-12 months old)

Exercise No. 17

Leg Stretching

Aim: To loosen up your baby's leg muscles; a good warm-up exercise.

Starting Position: Lay your baby on his back.

1 Holding your baby's ankles, cross his left leg over his right leg, then cross his right leg over his left leg. *Repetitions:* Repeat three to five times with each leg, alternating legs.

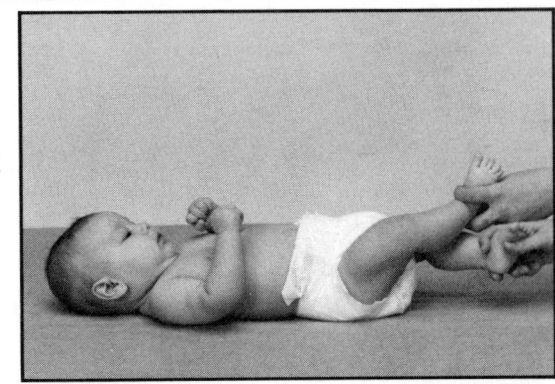

2 Raise his left leg above his head, then lower it. Raise his right leg above his head, then lower it. *Repetitions:* Repeat three to five times, alternating legs.

3 Holding onto your baby's ankles, slowly stretch his legs into a V one time.

PARENT/BABY EXERCISES (for babies 4-12 months old)

Exercise No. 18

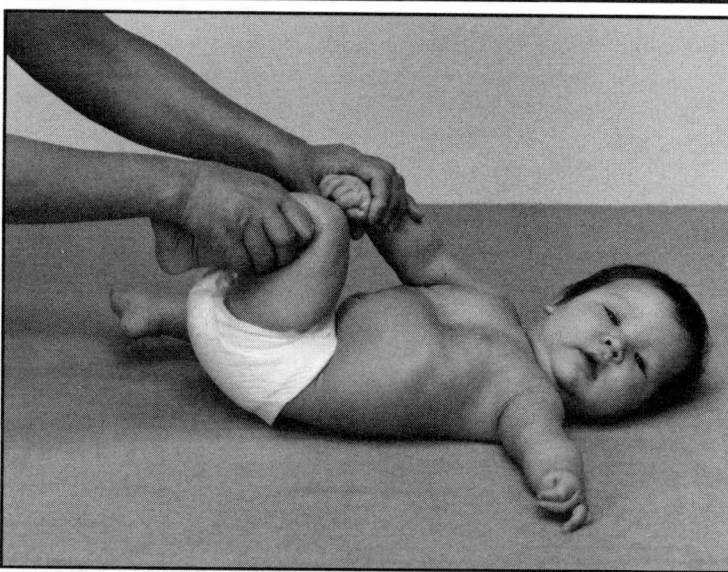

1 Raise her left knee while you bring her right hand down to slap her left knee lightly.

Knee Slappin'

Aim: To stretch your baby's body and improve her coordination.

Starting Position: Lay your baby on her back.

2 Raise her right knee and slap it with her left hand. *Repetitions:* Repeat five times on each side, alternating sides.

PARENT/BABY EXERCISES (for babies 4-12 months old)

Exercise No. 19

Baby Rainbows

Aim: To exercise your baby's entire leg; may help correct any tendency toward a "toed-in" walk.

Starting Position: Lay your baby on his back.

1 Raise his left leg slightly, then gently cross it over his right leg until his toes touch the floor.

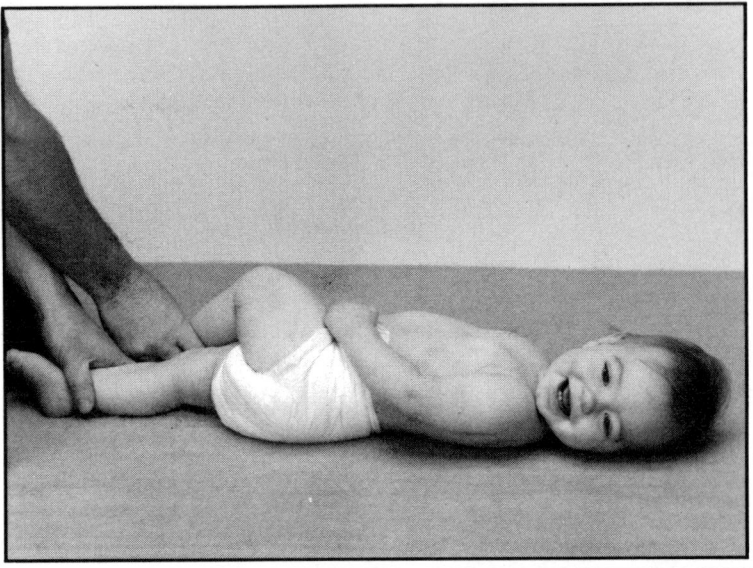

2 Roll his left leg outward to his left side, then return to starting position. Repeat with his right leg.
Repetitions: Repeat five times on each leg, alternating legs.

PARENT/BABY EXERCISES (for babies 4-12 months old)

Exercise No. 20

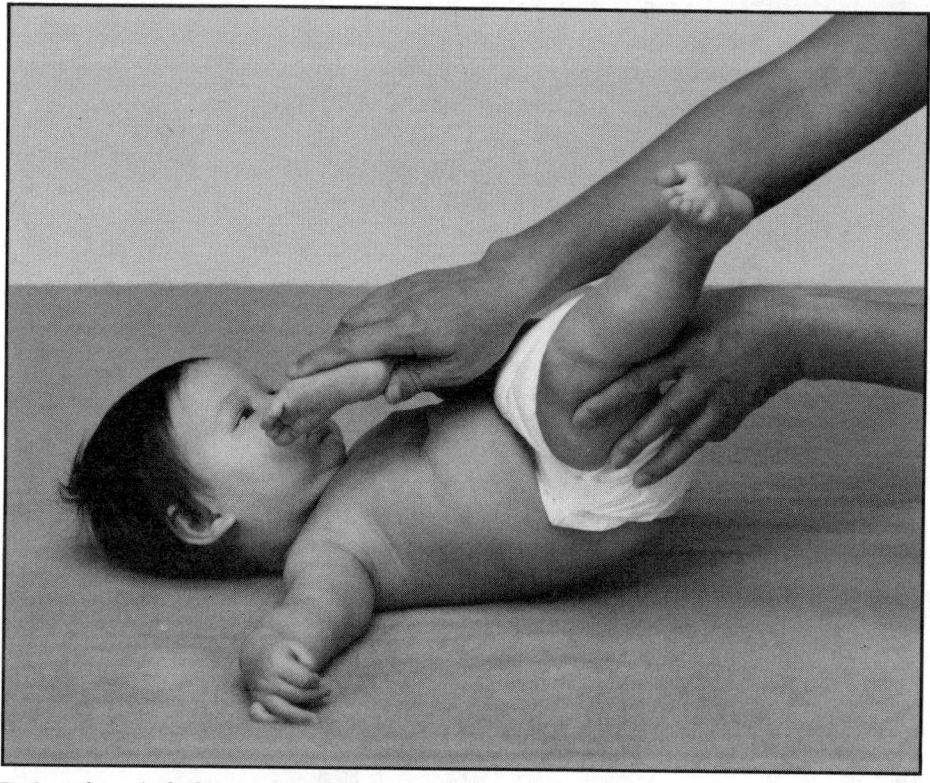

Touch Your Ear

Aim: To stretch your baby's entire body.

Starting Position: Lay your baby on her back.

Bring her left foot up, and touch the big toe of her left foot to her right ear. Touch the big toe of her right foot to her left ear. *Repetitions:* Repeat five to ten times with each foot, alternating sides.

PARENT/BABY EXERCISES (for babies 4-12 months old)

Exercise No. 21

Sitting

Aim: To prepare your baby for sitting, and to help develop the muscles he will use to pull himself to an upright position.

Starting Position: *Pull-ups:* Lay your baby on his back. *See-saws:* Sit on the floor with your legs apart and your baby lying on his back, facing you.

1 *Pull-ups:* Let your baby grasp your thumbs with both hands (Palmar grasp). Gently pull both of his arms upward, until you just begin to lift him off the floor.

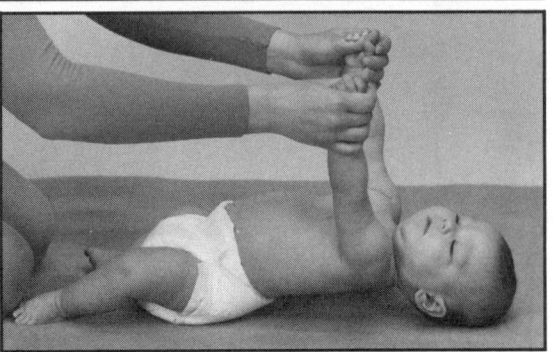

2 Keeping your hands very still at that position, allow your baby to pull himself up to your fingers.
Repetitions: Repeat two or three times.

1 *See-saws (sit-ups):* Bend your right leg in and push your baby's legs against your right leg so that his legs are bent.

2 Have him grasp your thumbs, then wrap your hands around his and gently pull him up. Let him back down gently. If his head drops back when you pull him up, STOP the exercise. *Repetitions:* Start with five; work up to thirty.

Note: When you do see-saws with your baby, say "up and down" to him as he moves, to help him recognize the concept of going up and down.

PARENT/BABY EXERCISES (for babies 4-12 months old)

Exercise No. 21

Sitting

Sitting on the Floor: Seat your baby between your legs, facing away from you, while he rests against you. As your baby gains confidence, move back little by little until he is sitting by himself. *Do not* prop him up. Try letting him sit in a beanbag chair while you watch him.

Sitting on a Stool or Chair: Do not support your baby's back; give him a chance to balance on his own. To encourage him to keep his back straight, move a toy from side to side while he sits. For fun, play finger games with him while he sits.

Aim: To help your baby learn to sit by himself and to encourage good posture.

Starting Position: *Sitting on the Floor:* Sit on the floor with your legs apart. *Sitting on a Stool or Chair:* Place your baby on a chair or stacked mats.

Note: Until he is strong enough and confident enough to sit on his own, a four- to six-month-old baby can sit with your assistance for up to half an hour a day.

PARENT/BABY EXERCISES (for babies 4-12 months old)

Exercise No. 22

Games on the Roll

Aim: To strengthen your baby's arms and legs for crawling.

Starting Position: Place a toy in front of a roll. Lay your baby on her stomach over the roll, holding her securely, keeping one hand on her back at all times.

Note: Use the *Strength Test* on page 167 to see whether your baby is ready for these exercises. Your baby should be at least four months old before you attempt Game #2 with her.

Game #1: Push your baby gently forward and backward for a minute or two. Allow the baby to use her legs to move the roll.

Game #2: Encourage your baby to grasp the toy on her own, allowing her to support her weight on her shoulders.

PARENT/BABY EXERCISES (for babies 4-12 months old)

Exercise No. 22

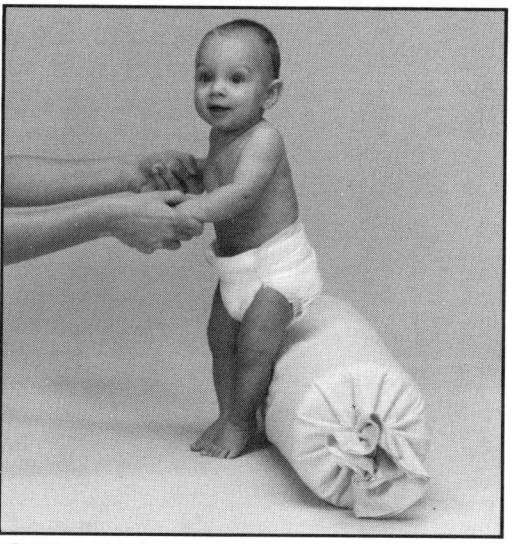

Games on the Roll

Aim: To improve your baby's balance and coordination.

1 *Game #3 (Sitting to Stand):* Let your baby sit on the roll while you hold her hands firmly.

2 Rock her gently from front to back, moving her gradually to a stand. *Repetitions:* Repeat two or three times.

Game #4 (Astride): Place your baby lengthwise on her stomach on the roll, holding her tightly at the hips or thighs. Rock her from side to side, allowing her weight to fall on her hand and foot on each side. *Repetitions:* Rock her three to five times on each side.

PARENT/BABY EXERCISES (for babies 4-12 months old)

Exercise No. 23

Crawling

Aim: To prepare your baby to support his weight on his shoulders and arms, prior to crawling.

Starting Position: *Pattern for Crawling:* Lay your baby on his back. *Wheelbarrow:* Place your baby on all fours, with his weight on his arms and shoulders. Hold his thighs with one hand while supporting his chest with the other.

Pattern for Crawling: Bend your baby's right knee toward his stomach and at the same time raise his left arm above his head. Return to starting position. *Repetitions:* Repeat five times on each side.

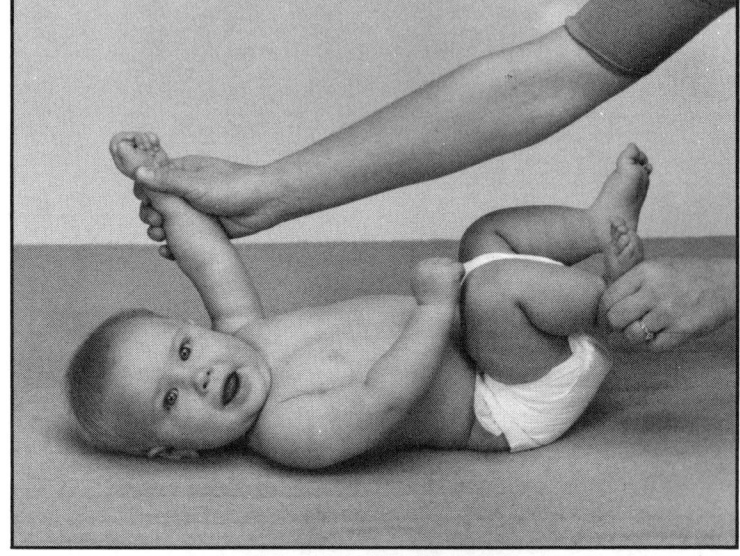

Wheelbarrow: Lift your baby's legs off the floor. Allowing him to support his own weight, "walk" him forward slowly on his hands for a very short distance. As he gets stronger, hold him at the knees—and, eventually, at the ankles—instead of at the thighs.

PARENT/BABY EXERCISES (for babies 4-12 months old)

Exercise No. 23

Crawling

Push and Creep: Place your left hand against your baby's left foot and resist while he straightens his leg. Immediately place your right hand on his right foot. Alternate legs as he moves along the floor. At first he may have difficulty freeing his hand from under him. Let him try to pull his arm out, but be ready to help him.

Aim: To strengthen your baby's legs and neck, to teach him how to reach, and to show him how to crawl properly.

Starting Position: *Push and Creep:* Place your baby on his stomach and tuck his feet up close to his body.
Fundamentals of Crawling: Place your baby on all fours in a crouched position.

1 *Fundamentals of Crawling:* Rock your baby back and forth (revving). Eventually he will catch on to this rocking motion and do it himself, in preparation for crawling. Try placing a favorite toy in front of him for encouragement.

2 When your baby is ready, help him move his left knee and right arm forward at the same time. *Repetitions:* Repeat with his right knee and left arm; alternate as the baby crawls.

PARENT/BABY EXERCISES (for babies 4-12 months old)

Exercise No. 24

Weight Lifting

Aim: To strengthen your baby's legs, develop her balance and eye/hand coordination, and teach her proper lifting techniques.

Starting Position: Stand behind her and hold her at the hips while she stands.

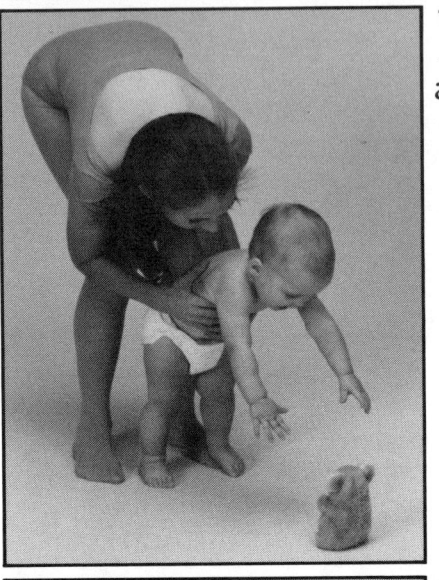

1 Encourage her to squat to pick up a toy or another object.

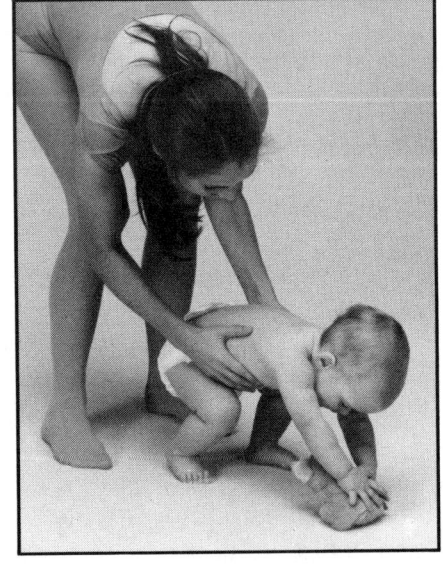

2 Return her to standing position. *Repetitions:* Repeat two or three times.

Note: Your baby must be able to stand on the floor fairly well before you attempt this exercise with her.

PARENT/BABY EXERCISES (for babies 4-12 months old)

Exercise No. 25

Walking

Crawling to Stand: Hold the push toy steady while your baby crawls up to it, pulls himself up, and uses it to walk. Eventually he will be able to push the toy by himself while you guide it.

Sitting to Stand: Hold the push toy while your baby pulls himself to stand up out of the chair. Allow him to use the toy to walk, holding onto the push toy.

Fundamentals of Walking: Allow your baby to walk with your assistance, making sure that his feet are flat on the floor and his body is bent forward slightly. Practice for a few minutes at a time, until he is walking alone.

Aim: To prepare your baby for walking by giving him confidence to walk alone and to help your baby develop a natural stride.

Starting Position: *Crawling to Stand:* Seat your baby on the floor beside a push toy. *Sitting to Stand:* Seat your baby on a stool or baby seat beside a push toy. *Fundamentals of Walking:* Hold your baby at the waist or hold his hands at waist level.

FAMILY TEAM EXERCISES

Exercise No. 1

Parents and baby will both benefit from the following exercises. Holding your baby while exercising increases resistance, which, for the parent, makes the exercises like exercising with weights. Start with a few exercises and increase the number as your family builds its fitness level. Try to add one or two a month to your baby's normal routine.

Roly-Poly

Aim: To massage your baby's back and loosen up your legs.

Starting Position: Pike sit. Place your baby across your legs, on her back.

1 Move your thighs up and down, alternating legs. *Repetitions:* Repeat three to five times.

FAMILY TEAM EXERCISES

Exercise No. 2

Side Benders

1 Bend to the left, then bend to the right. *Repetitions:* Begin by bending five times on each side, alternating sides; work up to bending ten times on each side.

Variation: Do the exercise with your baby turned around, his back against your chest. As he grows older, he may prefer this position.

Aim: To trim your waistline.

Starting Position: Stand with your legs apart, holding your baby in a tight hug, facing you.

185

FAMILY TEAM EXERCISES

Exercise No. 3

Sky Diver/ Parachute

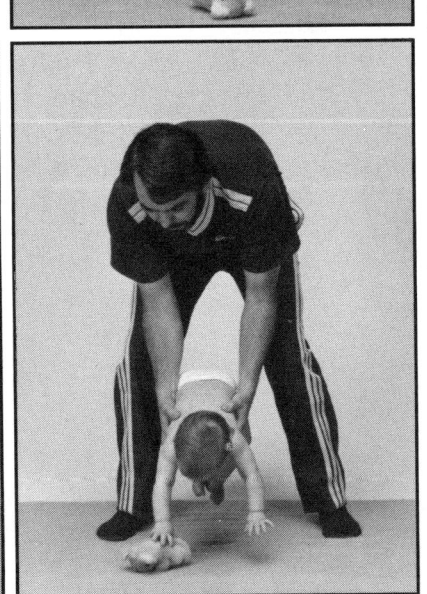

Aim: To develop your baby's Landau reflex and parachute reflex (see page 153 for more information on reflexes).

Starting Position: Stand with your legs comfortably apart and your knees slightly bent, with your baby sitting between your legs. Place a small toy on the floor about a foot in front of you.

2 Gently swing her back and forth two to five times.

1 Squat down and pick up your baby, placing the palms of your hands on your baby's chest/stomach.

3 Tilt your baby so that her head points toward the floor; she will try to reach for the floor (parachute). *Repetitions:* Repeat two to five times. To strengthen your baby's grip, let her pick up a small object from the floor in front of you and raise it off the floor as high as she can.

FAMILY TEAM EXERCISES

Exercise No. 4

Butterfly Rock

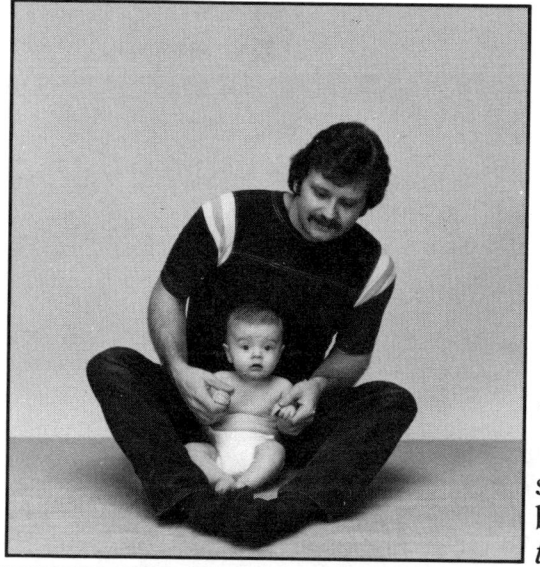

1 Gently rock back and forth, then from side to side as you support your baby in your lap. *Repetitions:* Repeat five times.

Aim: To strengthen your inner thigh muscles and tone your legs and waist, and to tone your baby's thigh muscles.

Starting Position: You and your baby face in the same direction in the butterfly-sit position, with your baby's back against you.

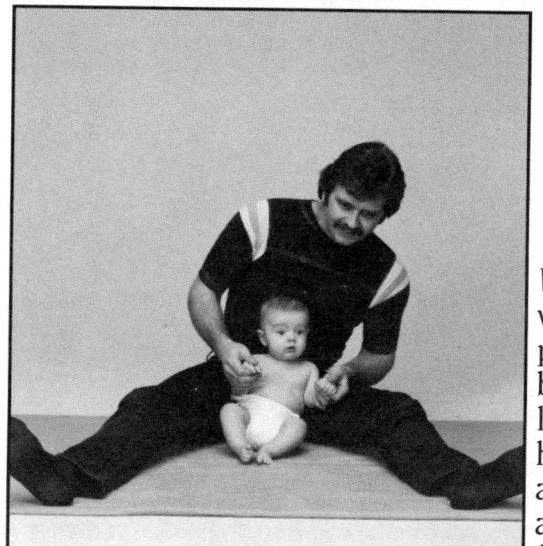

Variation: Try the exercise with you in a straddle-sit position. You can hold your baby's hands out at shoulder level in cross position to help him maintain his balance. *Repetitions:* Rock back and forth five times and then from side to side five times.

FAMILY TEAM EXERCISES

Exercise No. 5

Straddle Twist

Aim: To tone your baby's waistline.

Starting Position: Straddle sit, with your baby's back against your stomach, so that she is facing away from you.

1 Hold onto your baby's arms and gently twist her to the right, then the left, so that she moves from side to side at the waist.
Repetitions: Repeat five times on each side; work up to ten.

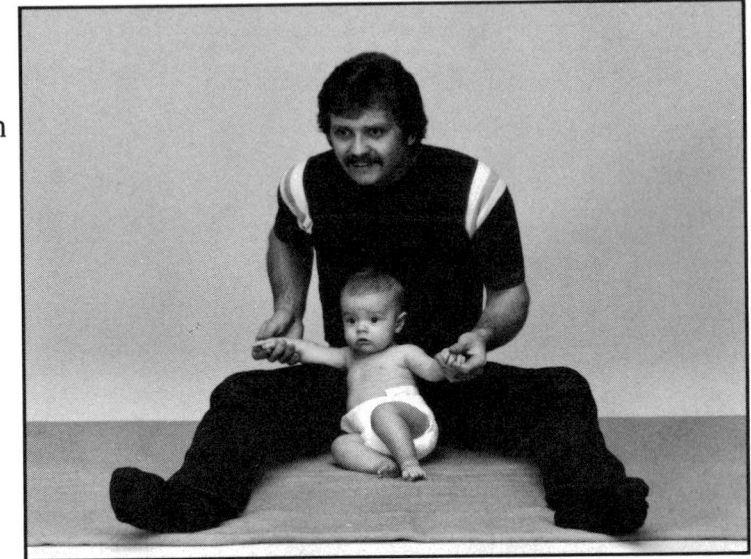

Variation (Row-Row-Row Your Boat): Hold your baby's arms and gently move them in a rowing or swimming position to the tune of "Row-Row-Row Your Boat."

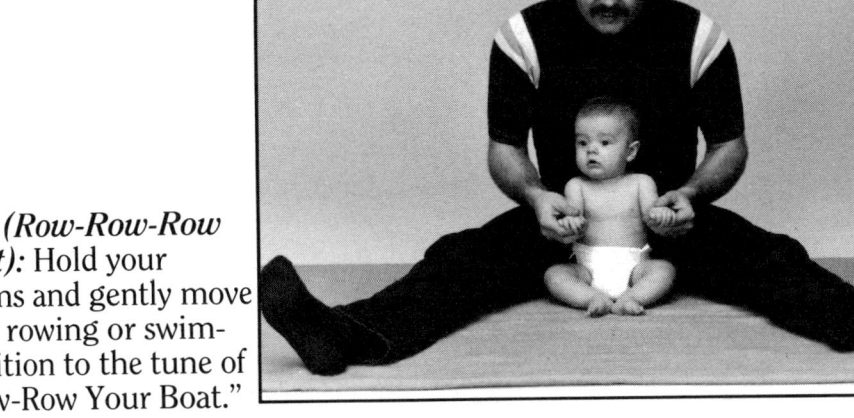

FAMILY TEAM EXERCISES

Exercise Nos. 6 and 7

"Walk" forward with your seat and legs; do not use your heels. "Walk" backward in the same way.

Ride Along
(team seat walks)

Aim: To tone your hips and legs.

Starting Position: Pike sit. Seat your baby on your lap with his back against you.

Note: For fun, put on a record while doing this exercise, and ride along with the beat of the song.

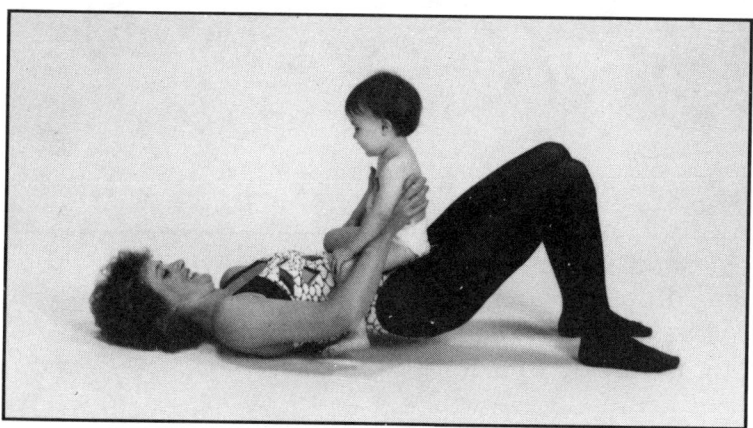

Raise your hips while you "tuck" your pelvis and pull in your abdominal muscles. Tighten your buttocks, then release the squeeze and lower yourself to starting position. *Repetitions:* Repeat five to ten times.

Ride 'em Baby
(team seat squeeze)

Aim: To strengthen your abdominal and pelvic muscles.

Starting Position: Hook-lying, with your baby sitting on your pelvic area facing you as you hold her around the waist.

189

FAMILY TEAM EXERCISES

Exercise No. 8

Porch Swing

Aim: To tone your waist and hips.

Starting Position: Hook-lying, with your baby sitting on your pelvic area facing you as you hold him around the waist.

1 Keeping your shoulders and feet flat on the floor, roll your hips, dropping your knees to your left, then to your right side. *Repetitions:* Repeat five to ten times, alternating from side to side.

FAMILY TEAM EXERCISES

Exercise No. 9

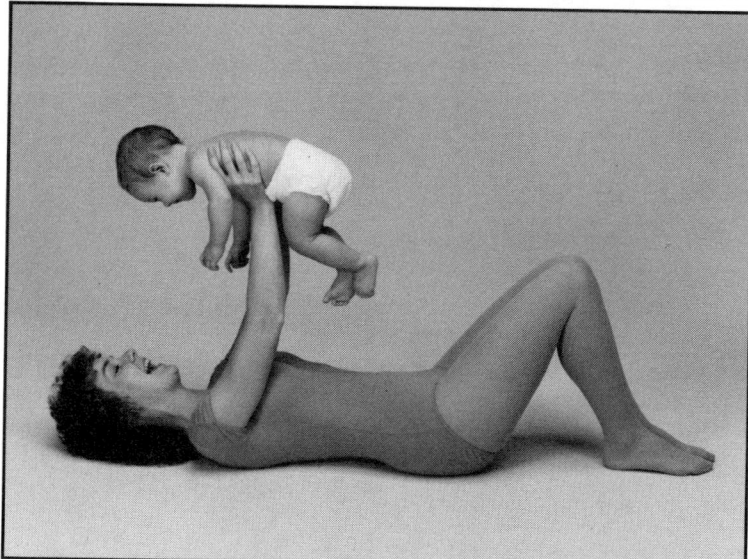

1 Holding your baby with your hands for balance, lift her until your arms are straight. Lower her to your chest. *Repetitions:* Repeat ten times.

Elevator

Aim: To strengthen your arms.

Starting Position: Lie on your back and lay your baby on your chest.

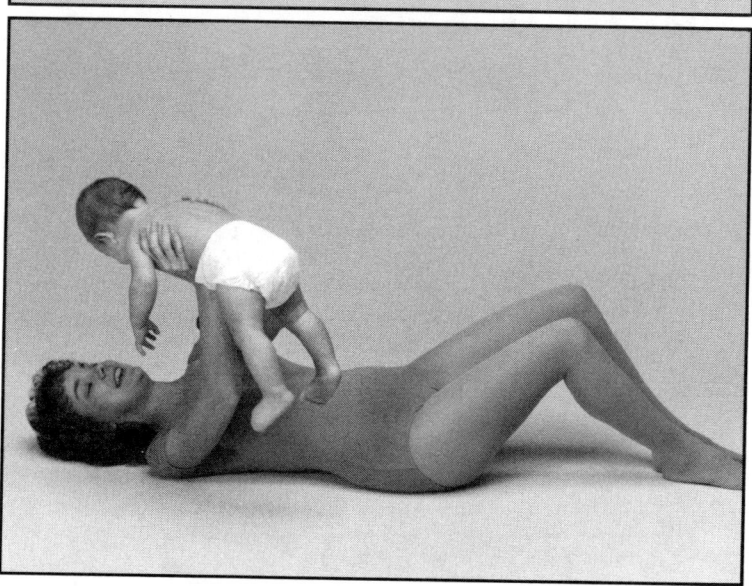

Variations: Holding your baby above your chest, move her in a circular motion, move her from side to side, and/or move her back and forth.
Repetitions: One time each way.

191

FAMILY TEAM EXERCISES

Exercise No. 10

Baby Curls

Aim: To strengthen your arms.

Starting Position: Stand, holding your baby in your arms.

1 Wrap one of your arms around your baby's legs and the other around his back, so that he is lying horizontally in your arms, parallel to the floor.

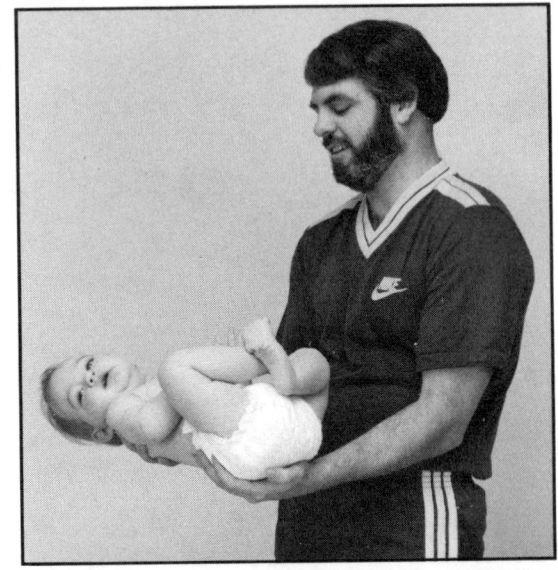

2 Slowly roll your arms open, then roll them back up. *Repetitions:* Start with two or three and work up to more.

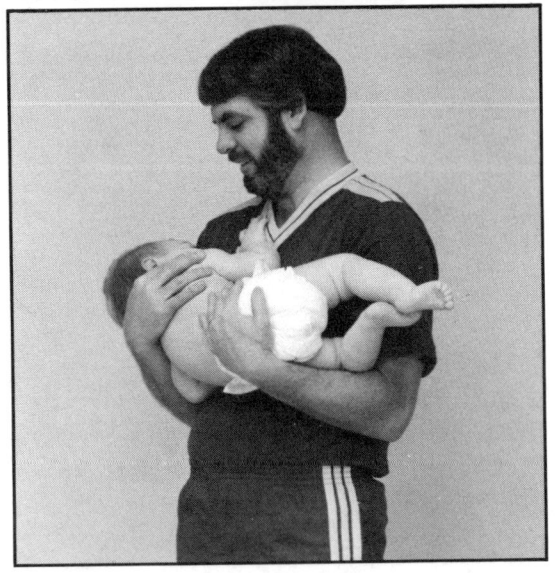

FAMILY TEAM EXERCISES

Exercise No. 11

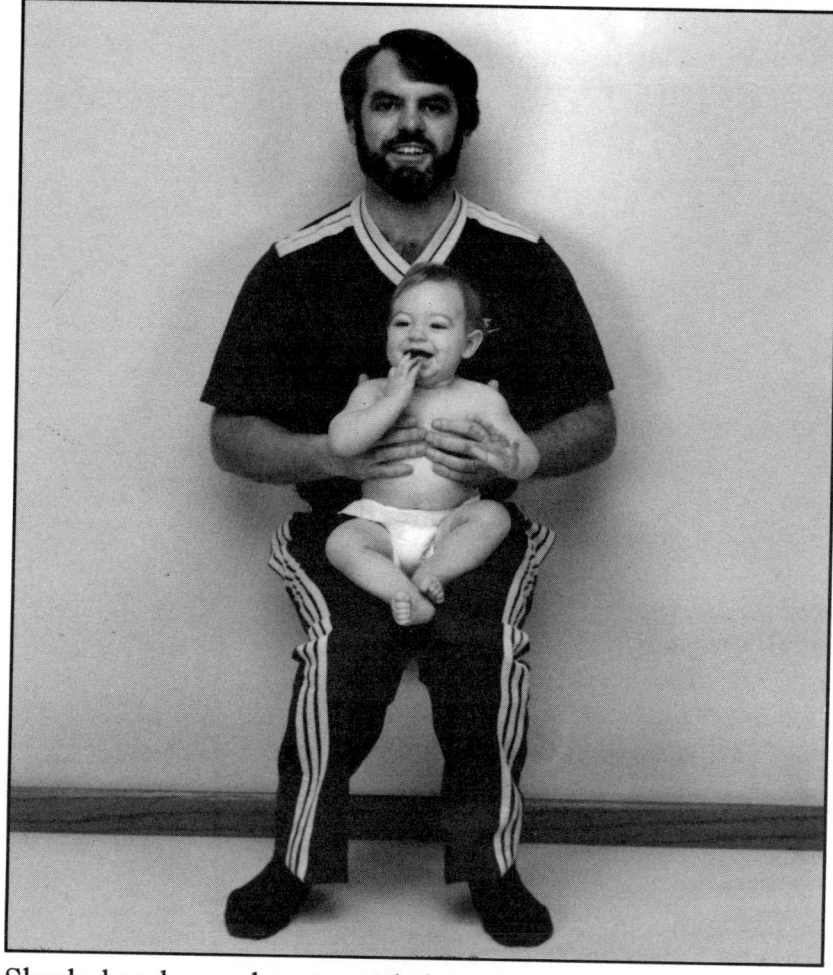

Skier's Sit

Aim: To strengthen your legs, abdominal muscles, and lower back.

Starting Position: Stand with your lower back pressed against the wall and your feet flat on the floor. Hold your baby with her back against your chest.

Slowly bend your knees until they are at approximately a ninety-five-degree angle to the wall (do not go any lower), as though you were sitting on a chair. Hold for five seconds or more, then slowly return to standing position. *Repetitions:* Repeat two to five times.

FAMILY TEAM EXERCISES

Exercise No. 12

See-Saws

Aim: To strengthen your baby's chest, hands, and arms.

Starting Position: *For babies two to four months old:* Hook-lying. *For babies four to twelve months old:* Straddle sit with your baby sitting on the floor between your legs, facing you.

For babies two to four months old: Seat your baby on your stomach with his back against your thighs, facing you. Hold your baby's hands as you do sit-ups with him resting on your thighs. *Repetitions:* Repeat five to ten times.

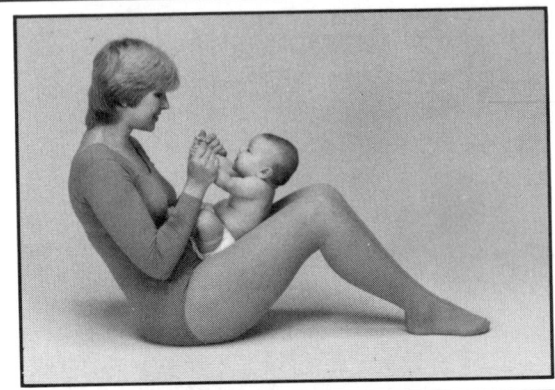

1. *For babies four to twelve months old:* Lay your baby on his back. Bend your right leg in and push his legs against your right leg so that his legs are bent.

2. Have him grasp your thumbs (Palmar grasp), then wrap your hands around his and gently pull him up. Let him gently back down. If his head drops back when you pull him up, STOP the exercise; try again in a few weeks. *Repetitions:* Start with five sit-ups; work up to thirty.

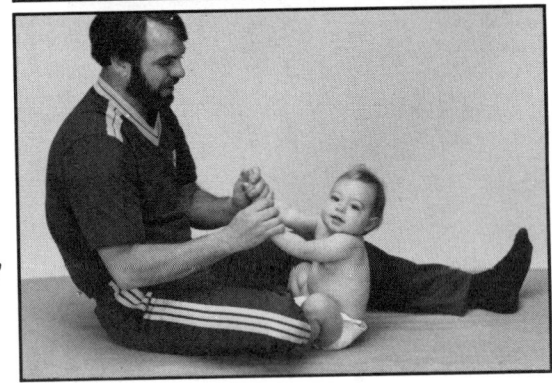

Note: Use the Strength Test on page 167 to see if your baby is ready to try this exercise. When doing see-saws, say "up and down" to your baby as he moves, to help him recognize the concept of going up and down.

FAMILY TEAM EXERCISES

Exercise No. 13

Jump-Ups: Seat your baby on your shins, facing you and holding hands. Your head and shoulders will be slightly off the floor, but be sure your lower back remains pressed to the floor. Let your baby kick off the floor while you remain stationary.

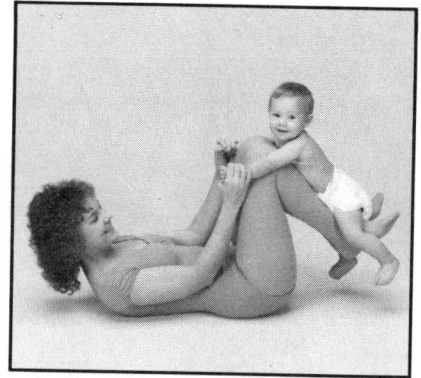

Knee Riders

Aim: To strengthen your abdominal muscles, shins, calves, and legs, and to strengthen your baby's legs.

Starting Position: Hook-lying.

1 *Giddy-Up Baby:* Start in raised-knee-rider position, with your baby up in the air.

2 Alternate bending and extending your legs so that your baby moves in horse-riding fashion, kicking off from the floor.

Slides: Sitting up with your knees bent, seat your baby on your knees, facing away from you. Holding her under the armpits, guide her down your shins to your feet.

FAMILY TEAM EXERCISES

Exercise No. 14

Tip-Toe through the Tulips

Aim: To strengthen your abdominal muscles.

Starting Position: Pike sit.

Note: Tighten your abdominal muscles while your baby walks up your legs.

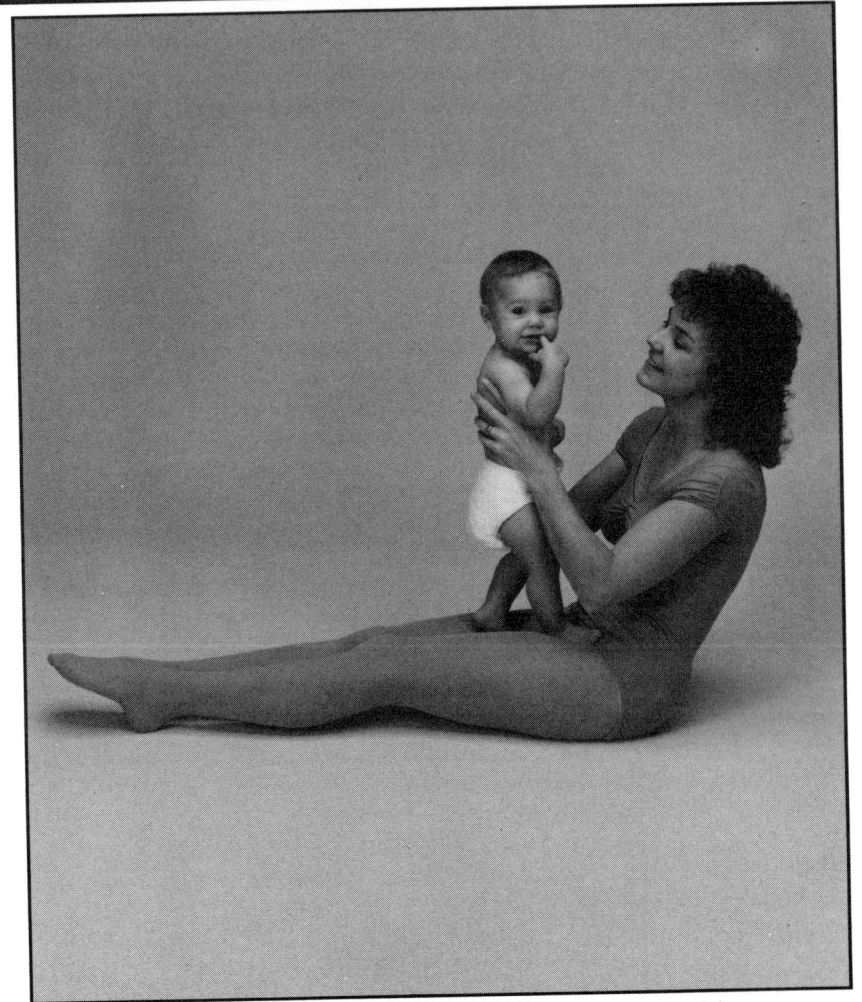

1 Stand your baby on your legs, facing you. Holding him under his armpits, allow him to walk up your legs to your abdominal area. *Repetitions:* Repeat two to three times.

FAMILY TEAM EXERCISES

Exercise No. 15

Peck and Kiss

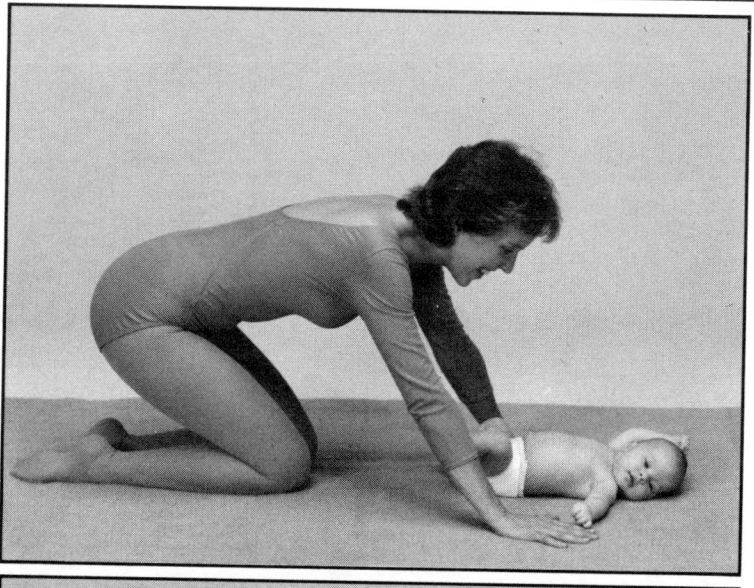

1 Rock forward, keeping your hands and knees in place.

2 Bend your arms and lower your face to your baby's face, then plant a big kiss on her cheek. *Repetitions:* Repeat five to ten times.

Aim: To strengthen your pectoral (chest) muscles, arms and shoulders.

Starting Position: Place your baby on her back on the floor and assume an all-fours position above her, with your hands near your baby's waist.

FAMILY TEAM EXERCISES

Exercise No. 16

Baby Sweeps
(for both parents and baby)

Aim: To stretch your hamstrings.

Starting Position: You and your partner sit facing each other in straddle-sit position, with your feet touching. Place your baby between you and grasp your hands to form a circle around the baby.

Rowing: Keeping your knees slightly bent, gently lean backward, pulling your partner forward from the hips. Try to kiss the baby. *Repetitions:* You and your partner reverse roles and continue "rowing" back and forth five to ten times.

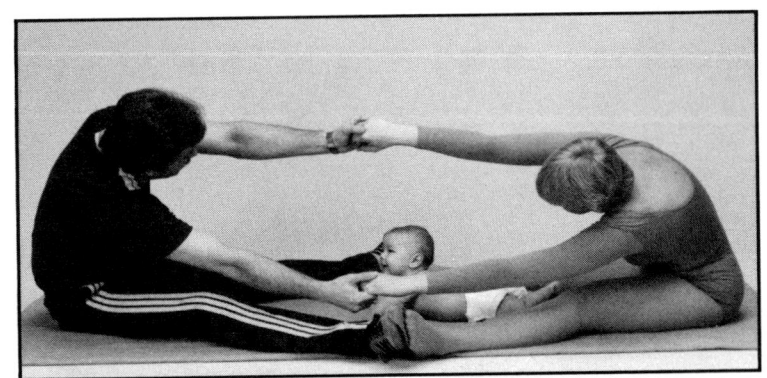

Sweeps: You and your partner "sweep" your upper bodies in a circular motion over your baby. *Repetitions:* Circle five times in each direction, alternating directions.

MAKE IT YOURSELF

Exercise Mat

Materials:

- One piece of foam rubber, 5 feet × 24 inches × 1/2 inch.
- Two sections of coordinating calico print fabric, each 1-3/4 yards long.
- 72 inches of bias tape.

Directions:

1. Cut the cotton fabric into 1-3/4 yards × 26 inches (use the darker color for the bottom side).
2. Machine-applique YOU & ME, BABY in a solid color on the top fabric, right-side out.
3. Place the right sides together (wrong sides outside and showing) and sew along both sides and one end, giving a 5/8-inch seam allowance.
4. Turn the fabric right-side out, stuff foam into the casing, and adjust for even distribution.
5. Make ties by cutting two 36-inch pieces of bias tape. Zigzag stitch down the middle to finish off the ties.
6. Turn the bottom seam allowance on the mat in 5/8 inch and topstitch the edges together, placing bias tape ties in the seam at both ends. Secure the ties into the seam.
7. Roll up the mat, tie it, and you're ready to go.

Note: To make a baby exercise roll, roll up the mat and tie it at both ends.

To make a baby exercise roll that involves no sewing:

A suitable roll for these exercises can be made from a purchased foam bolster, 7 inches in diameter and 18 inches wide. You can cover it with toweling or colorful, washable fabric tied with ribbons on each end. As your baby gets older, add towels to adjust it to fit. The baby fits a roll when he can touch his hands in front of him and his feet are slightly off the floor behind him.

MAKE IT YOURSELF

Little Beanbag Chair Pattern

Materials:
- 3-1/2 yards of 45-inch or 3 yards of 60-inch material.
- Heavy-duty thread.
- Pellets to fill the chair.

Directions:

1. General notes: 1/2-inch seam allowances; sew all seams twice.

2. Cut one 9-inch circle, two 18-inch half circles, and six main pieces (see layout design).

3. Take two main pieces, place the right sides together, then stitch them and press the seam open. Continue to add the main pieces in like manner, until all six main pieces are sewn together, then join the first and last stitched pieces and stitch together to form a completed circle.

4. Place the 9-inch circle on top, matching the tops of the chair. Stitch, fitting in place as you sew.

5. Press under 1/2 inch on the raw edge of an 18-inch half circle. Sew the wrong sides of the circle together, leaving a seam opening of 5 inches.

6. Place the bottom circle and stitch it, fitting it as you sew it to the wrong sides. Then turn the chair right-side out and fill it with pellets.

7. Slipstitch the opening closed, very tightly.

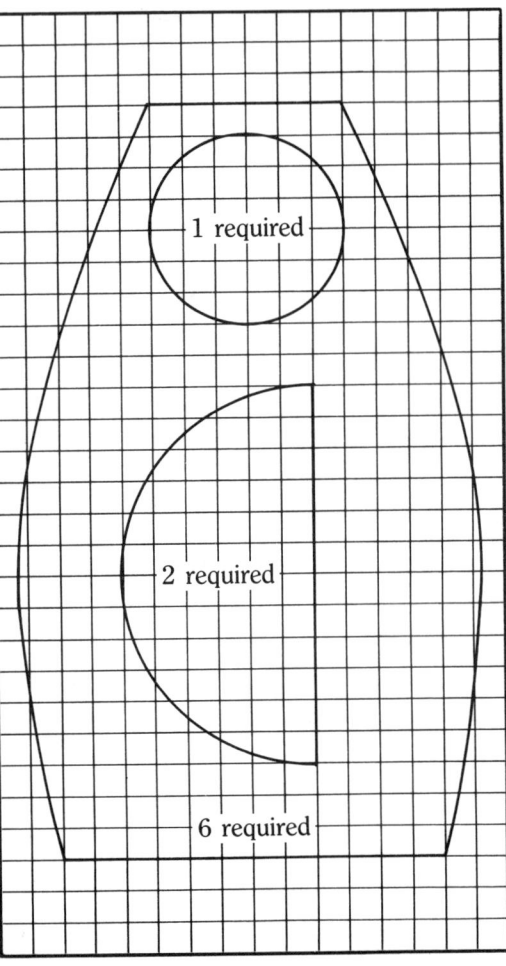

Pattern

1 required

2 required

6 required

1 square = 1½ inches

Appendix

Books

- Bing, Elisabeth. *Moving through Pregnancy* (Bantam).
- Levy, Janine, M.D. *The Baby Exercise Book* (Pantheon).
- Schneider, Virmala. *Infant Massage: A Handbook for Loving Parents* (Bantam).
- Simkin, Penny, R.P.T.; Whalley, Janet, R.N.; and Keppler, Ann, R.N. *Pregnancy, Childbirth, and the Newborn* (Meadowbrook).

Periodicals

American Baby, 575 Lexington Ave., New York, NY 10022.

Baby Talk, 185 Madison Ave., New York, NY 10016.

Growing Child/Growing Parent, 22 N. Second St., Lafayette, IN 47902.

Mothers Today, P.O. Box 243, Franklin Lakes, NJ 07417.

Parents, 80 New Bridge Rd., Bergenfield, NJ 07621.

The Physician and Sports Medicine, 4530 W. 77th St., Minneapolis, MN 55435.

Today's Health, American Medical Association, 535 N. Dearborn St., Chicago, IL 60610.

Organizations

American Medical Association
535 N. Dearborn St.
Chicago, IL 60610

American Running and Fitness Association
2420 K St. NW
Washington, DC 20037

Melpomene Institute for Women's Health Research
316 University Ave.
St. Paul, MN 55103

National Council of the YMCA of the USA
Director of Health Enhancement
101 N. Wacker Drive, Suite 1400
Chicago, IL 60606

YMCA of the USA, Program Resources
P.O. Box 5077
Champaign, IL 61820
(write for current catalog)

National Dairy Council
6300 N. River Rd.
Rosemount, IL 60018

American College of Obstetrics/Gynecology
600 Maryland Ave. SW, Suite 300 East
Washington, DC 20024

American Academy of Pediatrics
P.O. Box 1034
Evanston, IL 60204

APPENDIX

Pregnancy Primer

Condition	Possible Causes	Possible Solutions
Backaches	Poor posture, enlarging uterus, loss of abdominal tone, incorrect body mechanics, body weight distribution, change in center of gravity, muscle tension due to stress, lack of flexibility, history of back problems (pathological or congenital), previous injuries, overused lumbar muscles.	Get a firm mattress, sleep on your side, exercise daily, avoid lifting and twisting, use proper posture techniques, wear low-heeled shoes, do pelvic rocking on back and all fours. Use proper lifting and bending techniques—avoid lifting anything higher than eye level, and lift only reasonable amounts, i.e., a maximum of one-fourth of your body weight (this is particularly a problem for women who have older children who want to be picked up for attention). Practice the tuck and pull exercise: "tuck" your pelvis and pull in your abdominal muscles.
Constipation	Hormonal changes cause your intestines to become sluggish, and your growing uterus displaces the intestinal tract.	Drink plenty of fluids, especially water; eat high-fiber foods, green leafy vegetables, grains. Get plenty of exercise. Avoid soda pop, caffeine, and alcohol.
Dizziness and Fainting Note: Notify your doctor if visual disturbances accompany dizziness or fainting.	Increased blood volume from pregnancy, decreased hemoglobin, low blood sugar.	Get up slowly; flex your ankles and bend your legs at the knees before getting up. Wear support stockings to promote better circulation to the upper part of your body (especially the brain). Eat protein-rich foods, not just carbohydrates, in the morning.
Edema (normal swelling of the extremities or face; not to be confused with metabolic edema or toxemia)	Retention of fluid.	Increase your water intake, elevate your legs, rest, and exercise. Consider water exercise as an alternative to "on land" exercise.

APPENDIX

Pregnancy Primer

Condition	Possible Causes	Possible Solutions
Intestinal and Stomach Gas	Changes in body chemistry; physical pressure from the baby's growth causes decreased mobility of the intestinal tract, causing gas to form and the enlarging uterus to press on your intestines.	Avoid gas-producing foods; eat smaller, more frequent meals; and chew foods well. Exercise to increase intestinal activity—walking is especially good.
Headaches	Tension, stress, poor posture, poor circulation, diet, fatigue, eye strain.	Use total body relaxation techniques; take warm baths; try massage on upper body, neck, temples; do deep diaphragmatic breathing (don't hyperventilate). Stick to proper diet and use proper posture techniques. Get plenty of sleep (add ten percent to your normal sleep pattern, plus a nap in the afternoon).
Heartburn (uncomfortable burning sensation in the chest)	Acidic stomach secretions flow into your lower esophagus (most common in the second and third trimester). May be caused by the growing uterus pressing on your stomach.	Eat small, frequent meals; avoid alcohol, caffeine, acidic juices, spicy and gassy foods. Try proper diet selection. Change your position—try standing, sitting, lying down, or sleeping propped on pillows.
Hemorrhoids (varicose veins in the rectum)	Hemorrhoids are produced and aggravated by the pressure of the developing fetus. They may be aggravated further at the birthing stage of delivery, and by constipation.	Eat a diet high in fiber, do the kegel exercise, increase your water intake, do the pelvic rock exercise. Try a sitz bath or witch hazel compresses (to make your own compresses, take four-by-four compress pads, place them in a jar or dish, cover them with witch hazel, and refrigerate). If you are having painful bowel movements, try placing your feet on a stool when defecating; this allows you a better body position and will ease pressure.
Insomnia	Movement of your baby, shortness of breath, urination during the night, muscle cramps, emotional stress and tension, improper diet.	Use extra pillows for support, exercise, take warm baths, drink warm milk or tepid water before bedtime. Proper diet is very important (avoid caffeinated foods—coffee, tea, soda pop, chocolate).

APPENDIX

Pregnancy Primer

Condition	Possible Causes	Possible Solutions
Nausea and Vomiting (a temporary condition experienced by approximately 60 percent of pregnant women.) Note: Severe vomiting can cause weight loss and upset in electrolyte (i.e., fluid) balance. Consult your physician if this occurs.	Hormonal changes, emotional factors.	Eat complex carbohydrates in dry form (e.g., unsalted crackers, Cheerios).
Shortness of breath	Growing uterus, decrease in lung capacity, weight gain.	Do deep breathing techniques, change body position, exercise—especially walking.
Stretch Marks (may occur on the stomach, legs, breasts, and hips)	Heredity, loss of skin elasticity, rapid and excessive weight gain.	Keep your weight under control. Most women can tolerate the stretch from the developing baby, but excessive rapid weight gain may exceed the capacity of the skin to expand, resulting in stretch marks. You may wish to keep the skin lubricated with petroleum jelly or lotions; the best time to apply them is before going to bed. Never use petroleum jelly or lotion prior to exercise, because they have a tendency to hold in body heat.
Urinary Problems	The pressure of your uterus causes a kink or pinch in the ureters.	Increase your water intake. Do not do kegels; this could worsen the problem. Note: If this condition persists, see your doctor.
Varicose Veins (veins that have become enlarged and engorged with blood, usually in the lower extremities and/or rectal area. Varicose veins that appear or worsen with pregnancy often will improve after the pregnancy.)	Heredity, increased blood volume during pregnancy, which puts more strain on blood vessels. The enlarging uterus presses on the vessel that runs to your legs, causing slower return of blood from the legs and more strain on veins in the legs and perineum.	Elevate your legs, pressing your feet gently to the wall, several times a day. Wear support hose, especially when exercising. Avoid any binding hose, socks or clothes. Cool down after exercising.

Index

Abdominal Series 115-116
Afterbirth pains 83
Alcohol 4, 202
All Fours 16
Arm exercises
   postpartum series 103-106, 146-147
   prenatal 26
      series 48-50
Arm Positions 15
Arm Series 47
Arm Stretching
   for babies 0-4 mos. old 157
   for babies 4-12 mos. old 171

Baby Curls 192
Baby exercises 149-193
   for babies 0-4 mos. old 154-166
   for babies 4-12 mos. old 167-183
   tips on 149
   see also Names of individual exercises
Baby-Go-Round 63
Baby Massage 150-152
Baby Rainbows 174
Baby Sweeps 198
Back Arch 169
Back Tuck 16
Back Tucks
   after vaginal delivery 88
   postpartum exercise 117
Backache 202
   exercises to relieve 8, 35-36, 39, 56, 66, 74, 82
Basic Positions 14-16
Beanbag chair, directions for making 200
Bicycle workout 12, 136
Bicycles 163
   On Elbows 113

Body Positions 16
Body Relaxation
   postpartum 134
   prenatal 68
Braxton-Hicks contractions 11
Breathe and Lunge 46
Breathing exercises 17-20
   Alternate Nostril 18
   Invigorating Breath 19
   Postpartum 79, 85
   Simple Breath 17
      cesarean preparation 72
   Sniffing and Vitalic Breath 18
   Swan Breath 17
   Yoga Breathing/Stretch 20
Butterfly Press 30
Butterfly Rock
   family team exercise 187
   prenatal exercise 30
Butterfly Sit 14

Caffeine 4, 202-203
Calf Stretch
   postpartum exercise 109
   prenatal exercise 53
Cardiovascular system 5, 8
Cesarean delivery 71
   exercise routine after 78-82
   preparation exercises 72-77
   recovery from 78
Cheek to Cheek
   cesarean preparation 77
   postpartum exercise 123
   prenatal exercise 37
Compresses 203
Constipation 202
Cradle Stretch 127
Cramps, leg and foot
   exercises for relief of 75, 80, 87

Crawling 180-181
Criss-Cross 160
Cross Position 15
Curl-Ups 33-34, 143-144

Delivery 71-89
Diaper Change
   for babies 0-4 mos. old 155
   for babies 4-12 mos. old 170
Dizziness 21, 69, 202
Drugs 4

Edema 202
   see also Water exercises
Elevator 191
Exercise mat, directions for making 199
Exercise roll, directions for making 199

Face Exercises
   postpartum 102
   prenatal 22
Family Team exercises 184-198
   see also Names of individual exercises;
   Parent/Baby exercises
Feet Flexed 15
Feet Positions 15
Finger Massage 70
Flagpole 168
Flex and Extend 159
Flex and Flutter 76

Games on the Roll 178-179
Gas, intestinal 78, 83, 202

Hamstring Straddle Stretch
   postpartum exercise 130, 140
   prenatal exercise 61

Head Arcs
   postpartum exercise 101
   prenatal exercise 21
Headaches 202
Heart rate 8-10, 11, 54, 92
   target heart rate charts 9
Heartburn 203
Heel/Toe Rainbows 121, 142
Hemorrhoids 202
Hip/Knee Rotations 23
Hip Rock 38
Hip Roll 131
Hook-Lying 16
Huffing/Coughing 73
Hug and Rock 156
Human Relations 2, 71, 91

Insomnia 202

Kegel exercise 6
   after cesarean 81
   after vaginal delivery 84
   in relation to urinary problems 204
Kicks 161
Knee Bends
   after cesarean 81
   after vaginal delivery 86
Knee Cross-Overs 132
Knee Gliders
   postpartum exercise 133
   prenatal exercise 67
Knee Lifts 97
Knee Riders 195
Knee Slappin' 173

Lateral Straddle Stretch
   postpartum exercise 128-129, 138-139
   prenatal exercise 60

INDEX

Leg and Foot Toner
  after cesarean 80
  after vaginal delivery 87
  cesarean preparation 75
  prenatal exercise 44
Leg Circles 124
Leg Elevations
  prenatal exercise 69
Leg Extenders 40
Leg Extenders Variation
  prenatal 41
  cesarean preparation 76
Leg Lifts 108
Leg Raisers
  after vaginal delivery 89
  prenatal exercise 31
Leg Raises
  postpartum exercise 120, 141
Leg Stretching
  for babies 0-4 mos. old 158
  for babies 4-12 mos. old 172
Lifecycle workout 12
Lower Back Roll
  prenatal exercise 66
Lying On Your Stomach 84

Massage
  baby 150-152
  back, lower (prenatal) 66
  finger 70

Nausea 204
Neck Strengtheners 164
Nursing exercise 126
Nutrition 2-4, 8, 202-204
  basic food group servings 3
  vitamins 3-4

Oblique Curl-Ups 144
Open Pelvic Rock 42

Palmar grasp 153, 162, 176, 194

Parent/Baby exercises
  for babies 0-4 mos. old 154-166
  for babies 4-12 mos. old 167-183
  see also Family Team exercises;
    Names of individual exercises
Patterns
  baby exercise roll 199
  beanbag chair 200
  exercise mat 199
Peck and Kiss 197
Pelvic floor
  musculature of 5, 6
  strengthening of 92
  see also Kegel exercise
Pelvic Rock
  after cesarean 82
  after vaginal delivery 85
  on all fours 39
  on back 32
  Open 42
Physiology 5
  see also Posture
Pike Sit 14
Plié exercises
  prenatal 28
    series 55
  postpartum series 112
Porch Swing 190
Postpartum Breathing
  after cesarean 79
  after vaginal delivery 85
Postpartum concerns 13, 91-92
Postpartum exercises 92-134
  strength training 135-147
  see also Names of individual exercises
Posture 7-8, 202-203
Pregnancy Primer 4, 202-204
Prenatal concerns 1-13
Prenatal exercises 21-70
  see also Names of individual exercises
Pull-Ups 162
Push-Ups 125, 145

Raggedy Ann
  postpartum exercise 98
  prenatal exercise 27
Rainbows (Heel/Toe) 121, 142
Raise and Roll 35-36
Recti Diastasis 6-7, 11, 115
  self test for 7
Reflexes, baby's 153
Relaxation exercises
  parent/baby 154
  postpartum 134
  prenatal 68
Resistance equipment 12-13, 135-137
Ride Along 189
Ride 'em Baby 189
Rock 'n Roll 166
Roll to Side 165
Rolling to a Standing Position 16
Roly-Poly 184
Running guidelines 11

Seat Squeeze
  after cesarean 82
  after vaginal delivery 88
  postpartum exercise 114
  Team (Ride 'em Baby) 189
See-Saws 194
Separation of abdominal muscles
  see Recti Diastasis
Shoulder exercises
  postpartum 99-100
  prenatal 24-25
Shoulder Turns 62
Side Benders 185
Side Lean 111
Side Raisers 122
Side Sit 14
Simple Breaths 72
Sit Backs 58
Sitting exercise 176-177
Sitting Pelvic Stretch 57
Sitting positions 14

Sitting Tucks 118
Skier's Sit
  family team exercise 193
  postpartum exercise 107
  prenatal exercise 54
Sky Diver/Parachute 186
Smoking 4
Squats 45
Standing Thigh Stretch 51
Straddle Sit 14
Straddle Twist 188
Start-Up Stretch
  postpartum 96
  prenatal 29
Strength test 167
Strength-training guidelines
  prenatal 12-13
  postpartum 13, 135-147
Stretch marks 204
Stretch and Press 43
Swimming guidelines 12

Tailor Sit 14
Thigh Roll 59
Tip-Toe through the Tulips 196
Toes Pointed 15
Touch Your Ear 175
Tuck and Pull 8
  cesarean preparation 74

V Position 15
V-Stretch
  postpartum exercise 119
  prenatal exercise 64-65
Vaginal delivery
  exercise routine after 83
  hospital exercises after 84-89
Varicose veins 204

Walking
  for babies 4-12 mos. old 183
  postpartum 93
  prenatal 54

INDEX

Walking-Arm exercises 94-95
Walking/Jogging 110
Wall Push-Ups 52
Water exercises 10, 21-26, 28, 43-44, 46-55
  benefits of 1
  for relief from edema 202
Weight
  distribution of 4
  gain 4, 204
  loss through vomiting 204
  postpartum 92
Weight Lifting 182

Yoga Breathing/Stretch 20

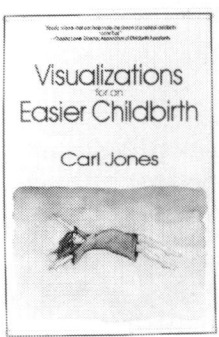

Visualizations for an Easier Childbirth
by Carl Jones

This book uses creative visualization and mental imagery to help ease pain and reduce stress during pregnancy. Includes 35 of the most effective visualization exercises ever created for pregnancy and childbirth.

Order #1330

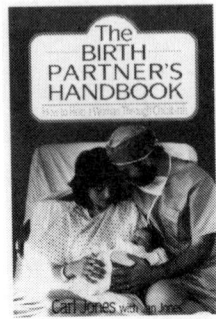

The Birth Partner's Handbook
by Carl Jones

Labor room companions can use this book as a childbirth class refresher course during the ninth month and as a bedside manual that details what to do when...Jones covers every potentially troublesome situation that may arise.

Order #1309

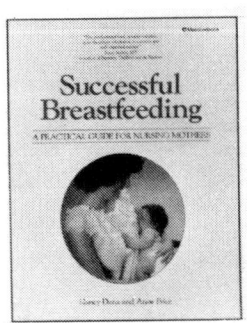

Successful Breastfeeding
by Nancy Dana and Anne Price

This the most practical illustrated guide for nursing mothers. It tells how to overcome the most common problems and complications mothers meet in breastfeeding.

Order #1199

Pregnancy, Childbirth and the Newborn
by Simkin, Whalley, and Keppler

The Childbirth Education Association of Seattle's illustrated guide to pregnancy and childbirth, nutrition, health, exercise, labor and birth, breastfeeding and new baby care. The most widely used prenatal training text in America.

Order #1169

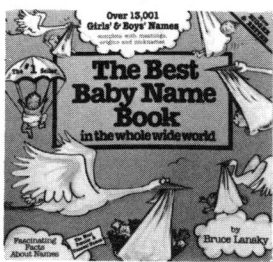

The Best Baby Name Book in the Whole Wide World
by Bruce Lansky

America's best-selling baby name book contains 13,000 up-to-date baby names It's the most complete, helpful, entertaining and gifty baby name book on the market.

Order #1029

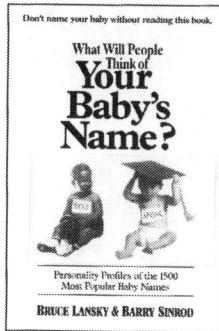

What Will People Think of Your Baby's Name?
by Bruce Lansky and Barry Sinrod

This revolutionary baby name book presents personality profiles of over 1,500 names so parents will understand what images and stereotypes are connected with each name—before they pick one. It's based on a national consumer survey of 7,500 respondents conducted by a leading market research company. And it's written by Bruce Lansky, the #1–selling author of baby name books, with over two million baby books sold.

Order #1270

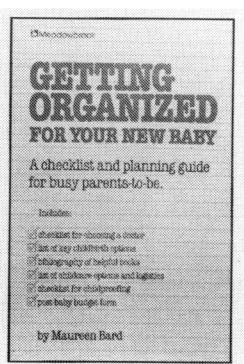

Getting Organized for Your New Baby
by Maureen Bard

The fastest way to get organized for pregnancy, childbirth and new baby care. Busy expectant parents will love the checklists, forms schedules, charts and hints because they make getting ready so much easier.

Order #1229

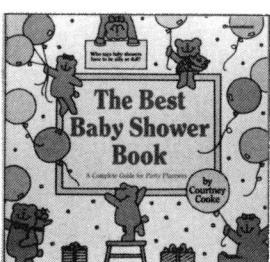

The Best Baby Shower Book
by Courtney Cooke

Who says baby showers have to be dull? Finally, a contemporary guide for planning baby showers that's chock-full of helpful hints, recipes, decorating ideas and activities that are fun without being juvenile.

Order #1239

Order Form

Qty	Title	Author	Order No.	Unit Cost	Total
	10,000 Baby Names	Lansky, B.	1210	$3.50	
	Almost Grown-Up	Patterson, C.	2290	$4.95	
	Baby & Child Medical Care	Hart, T.	1159	$6.95	
	Baby Talk	Lansky, B.	1039	$4.95	
	Best Baby Name Book	Lansky, B.	1029	$4.95	
	Best Baby Shower Book	Cooke, C.	1239	$4.95	
	Best Wedding Shower Book	Cooke, C.	6059	$4.95	
	Birth Partner's Handbook	Jones, C.	1309	$5.95	
	David, We're Pregnant!	Johnston, L.	1049	$4.95	
	Dino Dots	Dixon, D.	2250	$4.95	
	Dict. According to Mommy	Armor, J.	4110	$4.95	
	Don't Call Mommy	McBride, M.	4039	$4.95	
	Do They Ever Grow Up?	Johnston, L.	1089	$4.95	
	Empty Nest Symphony	McBride, M.	4080	$4.95	
	European Customs & Manners	Braganti/Devine	5080	$7.95	
	Exercises for Baby & Me	Regnier, S.	1099	$9.95	
	Feed Me! I'm Yours	Lansky, V.	1109	$6.95	
	First-Year Baby Care	Kelly, P.	1119	$6.95	
	Free Stuff for Kids, 13th Edition	FS Editors	2190	$4.95	
	Getting Organized for Your Baby	Bard, M.	1229	$4.95	
	Grandma Knows Best	McBride, M.	4009	$4.95	
	Hi Mom! Hi Dad!	Johnston, L.	1139	$4.95	
	Italian Without Words	Cangelosi/Carpini	5100	$4.95	
	Letters from a Pregnant Coward	Armor, J.	1289	$6.95	
	L.I.A.R.	Thornton, R.	4070	$4.95	
	Mother Murphy's Law	Lansky, B.	1149	$3.50	
	My First Years Photo Album		3139	$15.95	
	My First Years Record Book		3129	$13.95	
	Our Baby's First Year Calendar		3179	$9.95	
	Papal Bull	Sullivan, D.	4060	$4.95	
	Pregnancy, Childbirth, Newborn	Simkin/Whalley	1169	$10.95	
	Practical Parenting Tips	Lansky, V.	1179	$6.95	
	Rub-a-Dub-Dub, Science in Tub	Lewis, J.	2270	$5.95	
	Successful Breastfeeding	Price/Dana	1199	$9.95	
	Visualizations Easier Childbirth	Jones, C.	1330	$4.95	
	What People Will Think of Your Baby's Name	Lansky, Sinrod	1270	$6.95	
	While We're Out		3230	$3.50	
	Wordplay	Thiesen/King	2200	$5.95	
				Subtotal	
				Shipping and Handling (see across)	
				MN residents add 6% sales tax	
				Total	

Meadowbrook Press

YES, please send me the books indicated above. Add $1.25 shipping and handling for the first book and $.50 for each additional book. Add $2.00 to total for books shipped to Canada. Overseas postage will be billed. Allow up to 4 weeks for delivery. Send check or money order payable to Meadowbrook Press. No cash or C.O.D.'s please. Quantity discounts available upon request. Prices are subject to change without notice.

Send book(s) to:
Name_____
Address_____
City_____
State_____ Zip_____

☐ Check enclosed for $_____, payable to Meadowbrook Press
☐ Charge to my credit card (for purchases of $10.00 or more only)
☐ Phone Orders call: (800) 338-2232 ($10.00 or more only)

Account #_____

Visa ☐   MasterCard ☐

Signature_____
Exp. date_____

Meadowbrook Press, 18318 Minnetonka Boulevard, Deephaven, MN 55391 (612) 473-5400
Toll free (800) 338-2232